Musc   Therapy
for Geriatric Patients

atients has been
Geriatric Drug

The *Journal of Geriatric Drug Therapy* Monographic "Separates"

Below is a list of "separates," which in serials librarianship means a special issue simultaneously published as a special journal issue or double-issue *and* as a "separate" hardbound monograph. (This is a format which we also call a "DocuSerial.")

"Separates" are published because specialized libraries or professionals may wish to purchase a specific thematic issue by itself in a format which can be separately cataloged and shelved, as opposed to purchasing the journal on an on-going basis. Faculty members may also more easily consider a "separate" for classroom adoption.

"Separates" are carefully classified separately with the major book jobbers so that the journal tie-in can be noted on new book order slips to avoid duplicate purchasing.

You may wish to visit Haworth's website at . . .

http://www.haworthpressinc.com

. . . to search our online catalog for complete tables of contents of these separates and related publications.

You may also call 1-800-HAWORTH (outside US/Canada: 607-722-5857), or Fax 1-800-895-0582 (outside US/Canada: 607-771-0012), or e-mail at:

getinfo@haworthpressinc.com

Musculoskeletal Drug Therapy for Geriatric Patients, edited by Marie A. Chisholm, PharmD, and James W. Cooper, PharmPhD (Vol. 12, No. 4, 1999). *Discover the most up-to-date and unique assessments and treatments for postmenopausal osteoporosis, gout, and hyperuricemia. You will also examine geriatric rheumatoid arthritis and its treatment, such as the newest COX-2 inhibitors, that may provide safer and more effective relief than traditional acetaminophen therapy.*

Diabetes Mellitus in the Elderly, edited by James W. Cooper, PharmPhD (Vol. 12, No. 2, 1999). *Discusses the diagnosis and treatment of diabetes mellitus in the elderly.*

Gastrointestinal Drug Therapy in the Elderly, edited by James W. Cooper, PharmPhD, and William E. Wade, PharmD (Vol. 12, No. 1, 1997). *"This book is clinician-friendly. . . . Pharmacists caring for elderly patients will find the information contained within the book useful in optimizing their provision of pharmaceutical care." (Jeffrey C. Delafuente, MS, FCCP, Professor and Associate Chairman, Department of Pharmacy Practice, College of Pharmacy, University of Florida, Gainesville)*

Geriatric Drug Therapy Interventions, edited by James W. Cooper, PharmPhD (Vol. 11, No. 4, 1997). *Explores how interventions in geriatric drug therapy can improve drug adherence and reduce adverse drug reactions as well as contribute to improved disease state management in older patients.*

Urinary Incontinence in the Elderly: Pharmacotherapy Treatment, edited by James W. Cooper, PharmPhD (Vol. 11, No. 3, 1997). *"A very useful reference for clinicians working with incontinent patients in various settings." (Susan W. Miller, PharmD, FASCP, Professor, Department of Pharmacy Practice, Mercer University Southern School of Pharmacy, Atlanta, Georgia)*

Antivirals in the Elderly, edited by James W. Cooper, PharmPhD (Vol. 10, No. 2, 1997). *"The chapters are focused and full of useful detail. . . . Will help family physicians and those dealing with the elderly." (Canadian Family Physician)*

Antiinfectives in the Elderly, edited by James W. Cooper, PharmPhD (Vol. 10, No. 1, 1997). *"A useful resource for those treating common infections in the geriatric patient. This text should be extensively utilized." (Keith D. Campagna, PharmD, BCPS, Associate Professor, School of Pharmacy, Auburn University; Clinical Associate Professor, School of Medicine, University of Alabama at Birmingham)*

Geriopharmacotherapy in Home Health Care: New Frontiers in Pharmaceutical Care, edited by Steven R. Moore, RPh, MPH (Vol. 7, No. 3, 1993). *The contributing authors examine common problems and perceptions across states, both in medications and other programmatic concerns for the elderly.*

Musculoskeletal Drug Therapy for Geriatric Patients

Marie A. Chisholm
James W. Cooper
Editors

Musculoskeletal Drug Therapy for Geriatric Patients has been co-published simultaneously as *Journal of Geriatric Drug Therapy*, Volume 12, Number 4 1999.

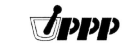

Pharmaceutical Products Press
An Imprint of
The Haworth Press, Inc.
New York • London • Oxford

Published by

Pharmaceutical Products Press®, 10 Alice Street, Binghamton, NY 13904-1580 USA

Pharmaceutical Products Press® is an imprint of The Haworth Press, Inc., 10 Alice Street, Binghamton, NY 13904-1580 USA.

Musculoskeletal Drug Therapy for Geriatric Patients has been co-published simultaneously as *Journal of Geriatric Drug Therapy*™, Volume 12, Number 4 1999.

Cover design by Thomas J. Mayshock Jr.

Library of Congress Cataloging-in-Publication Data

Musculoskeletal drug therapy for geriatric patients / Marie A. Chisholm, James W. Cooper, editors.
    p. ; cm.–(Journal of geriatric drug therapy; v. 12, no. 4)
    Includes bibliographical references and index.
    ISBN 0-7890-0789-4 (alk. paper) – ISBN 0-7890-0824-6 (alk. paper: pbk.)
    1. Musculoskeletal diseases in old age–Chemotherapy. 2. Geriatric pharmacology. I. Chisholm, Marie A. II. Cooper, James, 1944-   III. Series.
    [DNLM: 1. Musculoskeletal Diseases–drug therapy–Aged. WE 140 M9855 1999]
RC925.53 .M973 1999
618.97′647061–dc21
                                                                                                99-055307

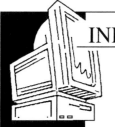

INDEXING & ABSTRACTING

Contributions to this publication are selectively indexed or abstracted in print, electronic, online, or CD-ROM version(s) of the reference tools and information services listed below. This list is current as of the copyright date of this publication. See the end of this section for additional notes.

- *Abstracts in Social Gerontology: Current Literature on Aging*

- *Adis International Ltd*

- *AgeInfo CD-Rom*

- *AgeLine Database*

- *Applied Social Sciences Index & Abstracts (ASSIA) (Online: ASSI via Data-Star) (CDRom: ASSIA Plus)*

- *Biosciences Information Service of Biological Abstracts (BIOSIS)*

- *Brown University Geriatric Research Application Digest "Abstracts Section"*

- *Brown University Long-Term Care Quality Letter "Abstracts Section"*

- *BUBL Information Service: An Internet-based Information Service for the UK higher education community <URL: http://bubl.ac.uk/>*

- *Cambridge Scientific Abstracts*

- *CNPIEC Reference Guide: Chinese National Directory of Foreign Periodicals*

- *Derwent Drug File*

- *EMBASE/Excerpta Medica Secondary Publishing Division*

- *Family Studies Database (online and CD/ROM)*

- *Human Resources Abstracts (HRA)*

- *Index to Periodical Articles Related to Law*

- *International Pharmaceutical Abstracts*

(continued)

- *New Literature on Old Age*
- *Psychological Abstracts (PsycINFO)*
- *Referativnyi Zhurnal (Abstracts Journal of the All-Russian Institute of Scientific and Technical Information)*
- *Social Services Abstracts*
- *Social Work Abstracts*
- *Sociological Abstracts (SA)*

Special Bibliographic Notes related to special journal issues (separates) and indexing/abstracting:

- indexing/abstracting services in this list will also cover material in any "separate" that is co-published simultaneously with Haworth's special thematic journal issue or DocuSerial. Indexing/abstracting usually covers material at the article/chapter level.
- monographic co-editions are intended for either non-subscribers or libraries which intend to purchase a second copy for their circulating collections.
- monographic co-editions are reported to all jobbers/wholesalers/approval plans. The source journal is listed as the "series" to assist the prevention of duplicate purchasing in the same manner utilized for books-in-series.
- to facilitate user/access services all indexing/abstracting services are encouraged to utilize the co-indexing entry note indicated at the bottom of the first page of each article/chapter/contribution.
- this is intended to assist a library user of any reference tool (whether print, electronic, online, or CD-ROM) to locate the monographic version if the library has purchased this version but not a subscription to the source journal.
- individual articles/chapters in any Haworth publication are also available through the Haworth Document Delivery Service (HDDS).

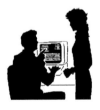

Musculoskeletal Drug Therapy for Geriatric Patients

CONTENTS

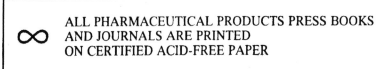

ABOUT THE EDITORS

Marie A. Chisholm, PharmD, is Assistant Professor of Pharmacy at the University of Georgia College of Pharmacy in Athens, Georgia, and Assistant Clinical Professor of Medicine at the Medical College of Georgia School of Medicine. She has published over 80 works concerning disease state management, pharmaceutical care, and pharmacy education and has presented on numerous occasions on disease state management topics including osteoporosis in the elderly. She teaches graduate and undergraduate courses in the pharmacotherapy management of disease states. Dr. Chisholm has received grants totaling over $1.2 million, most of these involving disease state management and educational studies. She has also received many teaching awards including the College of Pharmacy Teacher of the Year Award in 1997, the University of Georgia Richard B. Russell Undergraduate Teaching Award in 1998 and the Georgia Regents Teaching Award in 1999.

James W. Cooper, PharmPhD, BCPS, FASCP, FASHP, is Professor of Pharmacy Practice at the University of Georgia College of Pharmacy in Athens, Georgia, and Assistant Clinical Professor of Family Medicine at the Medical College of Georgia. He is the author or editor of 30 books and monographs, 10 book chapters, and over 400 research and professional publications. He teaches, practices, and conducts research in consultant pharmacy with geriatric patients in ambulatory and long-term care settings. The editor of the *Journal of Geriatric Drug Therapy*, Dr. Cooper is a board-certified pharmacotherapy specialist and a Fellow of the American Societies of Consultant Pharmacists and Health Systems Pharmacists. In 1981, he was a special advisor to the White House Conference on Aging. He is the recipient of numerous national awards for his work, and has received more than a million dollars in funding to support his research and service.

Introduction

Co-editor Chisholm and colleagues begin this book with a review of the assessment and treatment of postmenopausal osteoporosis. Osteoporosis, the most common skeletal disorder of the elderly, causes more than 1.5 million fractures each year, with annual costs to the U.S. health care system of approximately 14 billion dollars. Over the last few years several new pharmacologic agents have been approved for managing osteoporosis. These agents are discussed in detail in this issue.

Marshall and Miller present a thorough discussion of osteoarthritis and its drug therapy. The American College of Rheumatology, American Geriatrics Society and American Medical Directors Association have all concurred that acetaminophen should be first-line therapy of degenerative arthritis in the elderly, yet the most common adverse drug reaction of geriatric patients in long-term care is for NSAID gastropathy. [1]

Marshall has also authored a scholarly assessment of geriatric rheumatoid arthritis and its treatment. The newest COX-2 inhibitors and disease-modifying antirheumatic drugs may well provide safer and more effective relief to this arthritide.

Wade and co-editor Cooper conclude with an approach to the management of gout and hyperuricemia in the geriatric patient. Important considerations of which agent to use as well as when the need for chronic prophylactic therapy may be indicated are covered.

Marie A. Chisholm
James W. Cooper

REFERENCE

1. Cooper JW. Adverse drug reaction-related hospitalizations of nursing facility patients: a 4-year study. Sou Med J, in press.

[Haworth indexing entry note]: "Introduction." Chisholm, Marie A., and James W. Cooper. Published in *Musculoskeletal Drug Therapy for Geriatric Patients* (ed: Marie A. Chisholm, and James W. Cooper) Pharmaceutical Products Press, an imprint of The Haworth Press, Inc., 1999, p. 1. Single or multiple copies of this article are available for a fee from The Haworth Document Delivery Service [1-800-342-9678, 9:00 a.m. - 5:00 p.m. (EST). E-mail address: getinfo@haworthpressinc.com].

REVIEW ARTICLES

Management
of Postmenopausal Osteoporosis

Marie A. Chisholm
Anthony L. Mulloy
Jasvir Singh

SUMMARY. Osteoporosis, a reduction in bone mass density, is the most common skeletal disorder of the elderly. This crippling disease causes greater than 1.5 million fractures each year, with annual costs to the U.S. health care system of approximately $14 billion. Osteoporotic fractures cause pain, disability, and, in some cases, death. Although osteoporosis is a preventable and treatable condition, many postmenopaus-

Marie A. Chisholm, PharmD, is Assistant Professor, University of Georgia College of Pharmacy, Department of Clinical & Administrative Sciences, Athens, GA, and Clinical Assistant Professor, Department of Medicine, Medical College of Georgia School of Medicine, Augusta, GA 30912-2450. Anthony L. Mulloy, PhD, DO, is Executive, Specialty Care Service Line, Veterans Administration Medical Center, Augusta, GA; Director of the Metabolic Bone Disease Center, Medical College of Georgia; and Associate Professor, Department of Medicine, Medical College of Georgia, Augusta, GA 30912. Jasvir Singh, MD, is a Fellow, University of Georgia College of Pharmacy, Department of Clinical & Administrative Sciences, Athens, GA 30602.

[Haworth co-indexing entry note]: "Management of Postmenopausal Osteoporosis." Chisholm, Marie A., Anthony L. Mulloy, and Jasvir Singh. Co-published simultaneously in *Journal of Geriatric Drug Therapy* (Pharmaceutical Products Press, an imprint of The Haworth Press, Inc.) Vol. 12, No. 4, 1999, pp. 3-20; and: *Musculoskeletal Drug Therapy for Geriatric Patients* (ed: Marie A. Chisholm, and James W. Cooper) Pharmaceutical Products Press, an imprint of The Haworth Press, Inc., 1999, pp. 3-20. Single or multiple copies of this article are available for a fee from The Haworth Document Delivery Service [1-800-342-9678, 9:00 a.m. - 5:00 p.m. (EST). E-mail address: getinfo@haworthpressinc.com].

3

al women with osteoporosis are unaware of their fragile skeletal condition until fractures occur. Early diagnosis of osteoporosis is possible by measuring bone density and by targeting those at greatest risk of developing osteoporotic fractures. Treatment with calcium, estrogen, raloxifene, calcitonin, or alendronate stabilizes bone density in the elderly and reduces the risk of fractures. This article reviews the current strategies for evaluation, diagnosis, and management of osteoporosis. *[Article copies available for a fee from The Haworth Document Delivery Service: 1-800-342-9678. E-mail address: getinfo@haworthpressinc.com <Website: http: //www.haworthpressinc.com>]*

KEYWORDS: postmenopausal osteoporosis, elderly, pharmacotherapy of postmenopausal osteoporosis

Osteoporosis, the most important skeletal disorder associated with aging, is a significant cause of morbidity and mortality among the elderly. It is estimated that osteoporosis affects 75 million people in Europe, the United States (U.S.), and Japan. Furthermore, osteoporosis is associated with 1.5 million fractures each year, with annual costs to the U.S. health care system of approximately $14 billion.[1-5] Fractures most commonly occur in the thoracic and lumbar vertebrae, the proximal femur (hip fracture), and the distal forearm (Colles' fracture).[6] Approximately 33 percent of women and 15 percent of men over age 65 will experience a hip fracture. Hip fractures are fatal in 12 to 20 percent of the cases, and in other cases may result in long-term nursing home care.[7,8] As the population continues to age, the cost of treating osteoporosis and its associated complications are predicted to double over the next 30 years.[9]

PATHOPHYSIOLOGY

The two most common types of osteoporosis are type I (postmenopausal) and type II (senile). Type I osteoporosis, the most prevalent form, is characterized by a drastic decline in bone mass during the first five years of menopause and a slower rate of bone loss in subsequent years. Type II osteoporosis is characterized by a gradual, age-related loss of bone in women and men over the age of 70 years. Other forms of osteoporosis include idiopathic juvenile osteoporosis and osteoporosis secondary to other conditions which include early oophorectomy, hypogonadism, Cushing's syndrome, gastrectomy, hyperthyroidism, hemiplegia, and with the use of glucocorticoid and anticonvulsant agents.[1,2,6,7] In addition to menopausal-associated hormonal changes, other risk factors for osteoporosis have been identified. Major risk factors for osteoporosis in women include low calcium intake, medical factors such as thyroid disease, and lifestyle factors such as inactivity and cigarette smoking. See Tables 1 and 2 for a listing of factors and drugs that are associated with a reduction in bone mass density.

In osteoporosis, osteoclasts excavate cavities in bone that bone-forming cells, the osteoblasts, are unable to fully reconstitute.[10,11] Accelerated bone turnover magnifies this bone loss. Histologically,

---

TABLE 1. Risk Factors for Osteoporosis in Postmenopausal Women

Diet
Low calcium intake
Excessive caffeine intake
Scurvy

Endocrine Diseases
Addison disease
Cushing syndrome
Thyrotoxicosis

Environmental Factors/Social Factors
Cigarette smoking
Excessive use of alcohol
Low exposure to sunlight
Physical inactivity

Gastrointestinal Disorders
Malabsorption syndromes (e.g., Celiac disease, Crohn's disease)
Gastric and small bowel resection
Chronic liver disease (e.g., primary biliary disease)

Hereditary Factor
First degree relative with osteoporosis or a low trauma fracture
Short stature
Small body frame

Menstrual History
Early menopause (before the age of 45 years)
History of amenorrhea

Racial Factors
Asian women
Caucasian

Rheumatic Disorders
Ankylosing arthritis
Rheumatic arthritis

References[3,21,58]

TABLE 2. Common Drugs Associated with Lowering Bone Mass

Anticoagulants (e.g., heparin, warfarin)
Antiepileptics (e.g., phenytoin)
Chemotherapeutic agents
Glucocorticoids (greater than 7.5 mg daily of prednisone for over 6 months)
Gonadotropin-Releasing Hormone Agonists (prolong use)
Lithium therapy (long-term use)
Thyroid replacement therapy

References[3,21,58]

osteoporosis is characterized by a decrease in cortical thickness and a reduction in the number and size of the trabeculae of cancellous bone (Figure 1).[12] Thus, the trabeculae become disconnected, leading to a loss of compressive strength and increased risk of fractures. Bone mineralization is not defective in osteoporosis. It is the production of the organic bone matrix that is defective. This important characteristic of osteoporosis distinguishes it from osteomalacia, a disease of deficient bone mineralization.

Peak bone mass is reached at about 30 to 35 years for cortical bone and 24 to 26 years for trabecular bone. Before menopause, skeletal mass is preserved because the rates of bone formation and resorption are approximately equal. In women and men, after the age of 50, there is a slow loss of cortical bone of about 0.3 to 0.5 percent per year. In menopausal women, an accelerated loss of cortical bone is superimposed upon this age-related loss. It is this decrease in the bone mass that is associated with fractures in the elderly and postmenopausal populations. Generally, men have higher bone density than women, and African-Americans have higher bone density than Caucasians. Loss of trabecular bone begins at an earlier age in both genders, but the loss is far greater in women. Over their lifetimes, women lose approximately 35 percent of their cortical bone and 50 percent of their trabecular bone, whereas men lose close to two-thirds of these amounts.[13,14] It is hypothesized that these differences may account for the lower incidences of osteoporotic fractures in men than women.

CLINICAL PRESENTATION

Osteoporosis evolves as a silent, relentless loss of bone with no obvious early warning signs. Therefore, many patients suffering from osteoporosis are not aware of their condition. Unfortunately, clinically apparent signs of osteoporosis are not present until a fracture has

FIGURE 1. Photomicrographs of transileal bone biopsies taken from a 20-year-old patient on the left and from a 70-year-old patient on the right illustrate the loss of cortical and cancellous bone with aging. The continuous network of cancellous plates typically of youth (left panel) is transformed into a discontinuous array of narrow, widely-spaced struts typical of the elderly (right panel).

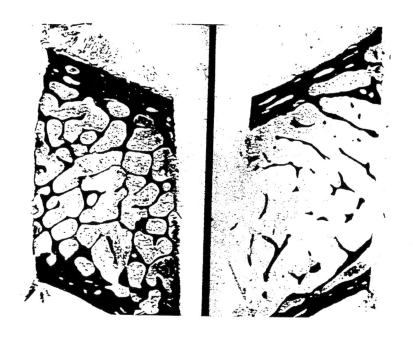

Reprinted with Permission.[12]

occurred with minimal or no recognized trauma. Acute back pain typically results from vertebral body compression fractures with deformity of the spine. The collapse of vertebrae can lead to spinal deformities such as dorsal kyphosis and dowager's or widow's hump. Severe kyphosis can result in a loss of 4 to 8 inches in height.[15] Postural slumping also contributes to this loss of height. In addition to fracture pain, a decrease in appetite, fatigue, and weakness may be present.

EVALUATION

Bone mass measurements are essential in the evaluation of osteoporosis. Although roentgenographic examination alone is too insensitive (estimates of the amount of mineral which must be lost to be recognized by a radiologist range from 20 to 60 percent), it is far from useless in the evaluation of bone loss.[1,16] Plain films of the hands may show subperiosteal erosions of the phalanges, characteristic of hyperparathyroidism; the skull may reveal the sharply demarcated, punched-out appearance of myeloma; and the pelvis may demonstrate pseudofractures suggestive of osteomalacia. Radiographs are also useful in detecting vertebral compression fractures.

Bone mass is best determined by dual-energy radiographic absorptiometry (DXA).[1] This technique increases image resolution and precision while minimizing the radiation exposure and measurement time.[16] Bone densitometry is necessary in all patients with osteoporosis to evaluate the extent and degree of bone loss, to establish the risk for fracture, to obtain a baseline with which to judge the efficacy of pharmaceutical intervention, and to diagnosis osteoporosis. The World Health Organization has defined osteoporosis as a bone mineral density that is 2.5 standard deviations below the mean normal peak bone density value in healthy adults.[17] In addition, identification of low bone mass may help asymptomatic menopausal women to make decisions about estrogen replacement therapy. A decrease in bone density of just one standard deviation from the normal race-and sex-matched mean peak bone density value increases the risk of fracture by 50 to 100 percent.[18-21] The cost-effectiveness of screening women to detect those at greatest risk for hip fracture has been described.[22]

TREATMENT

Considering the magnitude of the complications of osteoporosis, the best management is prevention. Nonpharmacological prevention measures include adequate calcium intake, weight-bearing exercise, discontinuation of smoking, reduction of heavy alcohol consumption, and limiting the use of osteoporosis-causing agents such as glucocorticosteriods (Table 2).

In the absence of hypercalcemia or nephrolithiasis, calcium therapy is safe and generally well-tolerated, except for complaints of constipation and gas. The National Institutes of Health Consensus Conference on Osteoporosis recommends an intake of 1500 mg per day of elemental calcium for postmenopausal patients.[23] Calcium supplements are best absorbed in divided doses given with meals. See Table 3 for the percentage of calcium in the various salts. See Table 4 for the common supplemental calcium products and the amount of elemental calcium that each product contains. Since calcium supplements bind with many drugs that may interfere with their absorption (e.g., tetracycline, phenytoin, and iron), it is recommended that these agents are not given at the same time as calcium but rather spacing them at least 30 to 60 minutes apart. The antiresorptive effects of calcium are not as great as those of estrogen-replacement therapy (ERT), raloxifene, calcitonin, and alendronate.

Vitamin D treatment may reduce fractures in the elderly due to its action in promoting intestinal calcium absorption and decreasing renal calcium reabsorption. Elderly patients may have insufficient dietary intake, decreased vitamin D metabolism to the active form, or low sunlight exposure. The Institute of Medicine recommends 200 IU daily of vitamin D.[24] The use of vitamin D is generally safe.[25] See Table 5 for common combination products containing both vitamin D and calcium.

Agents that decrease bone resorption act to diminish the imbalance between bone resorption and bone formation by inhibiting osteoblasts and reducing the rate of bone turnover. This effect is most noticed when bone turnover is rapid and the degree of imbalance is large. Gains in spinal density may be as great as 15 percent.[21] The most

TABLE 3. Percentage of Calcium in Various Salts

Salt	Percent Calcium
Calcium carbonate	40
Calcium acetate	25
Calcium chloride	27
Calcium citrate	21
Calcium glubionate	6.5
Calcium gluconate	9
Calcium lactate	13
Dibasic calcium phosphate dihydrate	23
Tricalcium phosphate (calcium phosphate, tribasic)	39

References[61,63]

TABLE 4. Common Oral Calcium Preparations

Trade Name	Type of Salt	Elemental Calcium
Alka Mints® 835 mg tablet	Calcium carbonate	334 mg
Cal Plus® 1.5 gm tablet	Calcium carbonate	600 mg
CAL-CARB-HD® 6.5 gm per packet	Calcium carbonate	2.4 gm
Calci-Chew® 1.25 gm tablet	Calcium carbonate	500 mg
Calciday-667® tablet	Calcium carbonate	266.8 mg
Calcium 600 mg ® 1.5 gm tablet	Calcium carbonate	600 mg
Calcium Carbonate 1.25 gm suspension per 5 ml	Calcium carbonate	500 mg
Calcium Carbonate 650 mg tablet	Calcium carbonate	260 mg
Calcium Carbonate 1.25 gm	Calcium carbonate	500 mg
Calcium Gluconate 500 mg tablet	Calcium gluconate	45 mg
Calcium Gluconate 650 mg tablet	Calcium gluconate	58.5 mg
Calcium Gluconate 975 mg tablet	Calcium gluconate	87.75 mg
Calcium Gluconate 1 gm	Calcium gluconate	90 mg
Calcium Lactate 325 mg tablet	Calcium lactate	42.25 mg
Calcium Lactate 650 mg tablet	Calcium lactate	84.5 mg
Cali-Mix® 1.25 gm powdered	Calcium carbonate	500 mg
Caltrate 600® tablet 1.5 mg tablet	Calcium carbonate	600 mg
Caltrate, Jr® 750 mg tablet	Calcium carbonate	300 mg
Chooz® 500 mg tablet	Calcium carbonate	200 mg
Citracal Liquitab® 2376 mg	Calcium citrate	500 mg
Citracal® 950 mg tablet	Calcium citrate	200 mg
Liqui-Cal softgels® 850 mg	Calcium carbonate	340 mg
Neo-Calglucon® syrup 1.8 gm per 5 ml	Calcium glubionate	115 mg/5 ml
Os-Cal 500® tablet	Calcium carbonate	500 mg
Phos-Ex 62.5 Mini-Tabs® 250 mg tablet	Calcium acetate	62.5 mg
Phos-Ex 167® 668 mg tablet	Calcium acetate	167 mg
Phos-Ex 125 ® 500 mg capsules	Calcium acetate	125 mg
Phos-Ex 250® 1000 mg tablet	Calcium acetate	250 mg
PhosLo® 667 mg tablet	Calcium acetate	169 mg
Posture® 1565.2 mg tablet	Tricalcium phosphate	600 mg
Rolaids® 550 mg tablet	Calcium carbonate	220 mg
Rolaids Extra-Strength® 1 gm tablet	Calcium carbonate	400 mg
Titralac® 420 tablet	Calcium carbonate	168 mg
Titralac Extra-Strength® 750 mg tablet	Calcium carbonate	300 mg
Titralac® suspension 1 gm per 5 ml	Calcium carbonate	400 mg per 5 ml
Tums® 500 mg tablet	Calcium carbonate	200 mg
Tums 500® tablet	Calcium carbonate	500 mg
Tums E-X® 750 mg tablet	Calcium carbonate	300 mg
Tums ULTRA® 1000 mg tablet	Calcium carbonate	400 mg

References [62,63]

TABLE 5. Common Oral Combination Products of Calcium and Vitamin D

Product	Contents	Elemental Calcium
Calcet®	Calcium carbonate 240 mg/Calcium gluconate 240 mg/Calcium lactate 240 mg/ Cholecalciferol 100 units	152.8 mg
Os-cal® 250 + D	Calcium carbonate 625 mg/Cholecalciferol 125 units	250 mg
Os-cal® 500 + D	Calcium carbonate 1.25 gm/Cholecalciferol 125 units	500 mg
Calel-D®	Calcium carbonate 1.25 gm/Cholecalciferol 200 units	500 mg
Caltrate® 600 + Vitamin D	Calcium carbonate 1.5 gm/Cholecalciferol 125 units	600 mg

References[62,63]

effective methods of using antiresorptive treatments occur when implemented as soon as susceptible patients are identified.

Estrogen, which works directly through estrogen receptors on both osteoclasts and osteoblasts, is very beneficial in postmenopausal women and is considered the drug of choice to prevent osteoporosis. It is approved by the U.S. Food and Drug Administration (FDA) for both prevention and treatment.[25] If started within the first few years after menopause, ERT can reduce the incidence of hip fractures by 50 percent. Even when delayed until osteoporosis is established, ERT significantly decreases the rate of fractures.[26]

Estrogen also raises high density lipoprotein (HDL) cholesterol levels and decreases low-density lipoprotein (LDL) cholesterol levels.[27] A follow-up to the Nurses' Health Study indicated a 60 percent decreased risk of major coronary artery disease for women on combined estrogen and progestin therapy or estrogen therapy alone, compared with nonhormone users.[28] However, a more recent trial suggested that oral conjugated estrogens plus medroxyprogesterone acetate may not reduce the overall rate of CHD (coronary heart disease) events in postmenopausal women with established coronary disease.[29] Further studies are needed to clarify the precise effect that estrogen has in reducing the overall rate of CHD events in postmenopausal women. Other benefits of ERT include relieving menopausal symptoms such as hot flashes and vaginal atrophy and dryness.

Minimum effective doses of estrogen are 0.625 to 1.25 mg per day of conjugated estrogen, 1 to 2 mg per day of 17β-estradiol, and 50 to 100 mcg twice weekly of transdermal estrogen.[30,31] Continuous estrogen supplementation is the regimen of choice in women who have had a hysterectomy; however, if the uterus is intact, oral estrogen can be given for the first 1 to 25 days of each month, and a progestin should be added to prevent endometrial hyperplasia. Medroxyprogesterone can be given for the last 10 to 14 days of each month at 5 to 10 mg per day. Alternatively, continuous estrogen and 2.5 to 5 mg per day of medroxyprogesterone prevent endometrial stimulation and usually lead to amenorrhea after 6 months of combined therapy. The addition of progesterone to therapy does not decrease estrogen's beneficial effects on bone.[32] No difference was found in the risk of breast cancer between estrogen alone and combined regimens of progesterone and estrogen.[33]

Tolerance and acceptance of ERT is limited by uterine bleeding, weight gain, breast tenderness, abdominal cramps, and skin irritation from the transdermal patch. In addition, fear of estrogen-induced breast cancer prevents many women from accepting the protective benefits of estrogen on the skeletal and cardiovascular systems.[34-36] ERT is contraindicated in women with undiagnosed vaginal bleeding, hypersensitivity to estrogen, thrombophlebitis, thromboembolism, known or suspected pregnancy, history of breast or endometrial cancer, and estrogen-dependent tumors.

Raloxifene, a mixed estrogen agonist and antagonist, is the first selective estrogen receptor modulator (SERM) approved by the FDA for the prevention of postmenopausal osteoporosis. Raloxifene has an estrogen agonist effect on bone and an antagonistic effect on both the breast and the uterus. This agent works by estrogen binding to reduce resorption of bone and decrease overall bone turnover. Trials have demonstrated that raloxifene decreases bone resorption and increases bone mass density.[37,38] Interim analysis of the incidence of fractures in the Multiple Outcomes of Raloxifene Evaluation (MORE) study of osteoporotic postmenopausal women showed that raloxifene reduced the risk of a vertebral fracture by approximately 50 percent compared to placebo.[39] Similar to estrogen, raloxifene decreases total and LDL cholesterol levels[40], and unlike estrogen, it has no effect on breast and uterine tissues. Raloxifene is contraindicated in pregnancy and patients who have a history of venous thrombosis or pulmonary embolism. The dose of raloxifene is 60 mg daily. At present, the long term effects of raloxifene on bone mineral density are not known.

Salmon calcitonin is a potent antiresorptive agent that is believed to act directly on osteoclasts. In addition to having effects on bone resorption, calcitonin may enhance osteoblastic bone formation.[41] Calcitonin, given at 100 IU daily or every other day (administered by subcutaneous or intramuscular injection) or 200 IU per day applied intranasally, has been shown to be effective in treating osteoporosis, reducing fractures and increasing vertebral bone density.[42-43] Calcitonin may have analgesic properties that facilitate mobilization of patients with fractures. Calcitonin is a good choice for the treatment of osteoporosis in postmenopausal women who will not or cannot take estrogen, in elderly patients with painful crush fractures, and in patients receiving long-term glucocorticoid treatment.[44] When administering calcitonin nasal spray, it is important that patients alternate nostrils daily. Calcitonin nasal spray should be stored in a refrigerator between 2-8°C (36-47°F), and once the bottle has been opened, it should be stored at room temperature. Injectable calcitonin should be refrigerated at all times. Calcitonin is relatively well-tolerated, with the most common adverse effect being mild to moderate gastrointestinal discomfort and flushing. Common adverse effects associated with nasally administered calcitonin include rhinitis, nasal symptoms (e.g., irritation and redness), and epistaxis. A skin-testing protocol is available from the manufacturer for patients with a suspected sensitivity to calcitonin.

Bisphosphonates are carbon-substituted analogues of pyrophosphate that are potent inhibitors of bone resorption. Bisphosphonates exert their action by adsorbing to skeletal hydroxyapatite. Once ingested by osteoclasts, bisphosphonates inhibit the vigor and viability of these bone-resorbing cells. These agents are retained in the bones for many years. Currently, alendronate sodium is the only bisphosphonate that is FDA-approved for the prevention and treatment of osteoporosis in the U.S.

The oral absorption of alendronate is very low and is estimated to be approximately 0.5 to 1.0 percent.[45-46] Administering alendronate with food can decrease the oral bioavailability by 40 percent; therefore, the current recommendation is to take alendronate after an overnight fast with water, and wait at least 30 minutes after taking the medication before eating. Patients should be instructed to take alendronate with 6 to 8 ounces of water and not to lie down for at least 30 minutes following administration to facilitate delivery of the medication to the stomach and reduce the potential for esophageal irritation.

Bone uptake accounts for approximately 40 to 60 percent of the dose, with uptake being greatest in active bone turnover sites.[45-47]

Alendronate increases bone mineral density and decreases fracture rates.[47-55] In addition, alendronate has not been found to cause a mineralization defect that may increase the risk of fractures. The recommended dosage of 10 mg per day of alendronate for treatment of postmenopausal osteoporosis was well-tolerated in the clinical studies, with the most common reported adverse effect being gastrointestinal discomfort and upset. The 5 mg daily dose of alendronate has been recently approved by the FDA for the prevention of postmenopausal osteoporosis.[56,57] Alendronate should not be used in patients with renal insufficiency (creatinine clearance < 35 ml/min), patients with hypocalcemia, patients with esophageal abnormalities or patients who are unable to sit or stand upright for 30 minutes. Long-term safety of the use of bisphosphonates for the treatment of osteoporosis remains unknown. Nevertheless, alendronate represents a promising approach to managing this disease.

THERAPEUTIC OPTIONS

Women who are at increased risk for osteoporotic fracture should be treated. This includes women who have already sustained a fracture with no or very little trauma and those who have a low bone density with or without other risk factors for osteoporosis.[58]

Patients with acute pain secondary to an osteoporotic vertebral fracture require bed rest and adequate analgesics. For additional pain relief, calcitonin may be used because of its analgesic properties as well as its antiresorptive properties. Patients should be taught to avoid sudden movements and lifting of heavy objects that might cause strain on the back resulting in vertebral fracture. After fractures have healed, a supervised exercise program that includes weight bearing exercises such as walking may be helpful in preventing further skeletal loss. Exercise also improves flexibility, strength, and coordination and may help decrease the risk of falls in the elderly.

In the elderly, fall prevention strategies, through evaluation of medications and a safe environment, are extremely important to reducing the impact of osteoporosis. Reduction of preventable risk factors such as limiting caffeine consumption associated with osteoporosis should also be considered. Due to increased risk of falling and causing fractures, limited use of sedative medications is strongly recommended.[59] Calcium intake should be maintained between 1000 mg to 1500 mg per day of elementary calcium for postmenopausal patients. Because alcohol and smoking have toxic effects on osteoblast and increase the risk for developing osteoporosis by twofold, excessive consumption of alcohol should be avoided along with a reduction in smoking.

It is important to individualize the pharmacological prevention and treatment of osteoporosis in each woman. Estrogen replacement is the treatment of choice for the prevention and treatment of osteoporosis in the postmenopausal population. In women under the age of 75 years, a minimum of seven years of estrogen use was required to improve bone mass density, compared to women who did not take estrogen. However, seven years of ERT had little effect on bone mass density in women over 75 years of age.[60] Thus, long-term and possibly indefinite use of ERT is recommended for maximal benefits. Alendronate, raloxifene, and calcitonin are alternatives to estrogen replacement and should be considered in those women who are not candidates for ERT (refer to Table 6). Vitamin D treatment may be prescribed for "housebound" or "institutionalized" patients with reduced sun exposure.

TABLE 6. Common Products Used in the Management of Postmenopausal Osteoporosis

Product	Indication	Recommended Daily Dosage
Alendronate–Fosamax®	Prevention/Treatment	5 mg 10 mg
Calcitonin–Miacalcin®[1]	Treatment	200 iu intranasally
Calcitonin–Calcimar® and Miacalcin®[2]	Treatment	100 iu injection
Conjugated estrogen–Premarin®	Prevention/Treatment	0.625 mg
Estropiate–Ogen®	Prevention/Treatment	0.75 mg
Ethinyl estradiol–Estinyl®	Prevention/Treatment	0.02 mg
Estradiol–Estrace®	Prevention/Treatment	1 mg
Raloxifene–Evista®	Prevention	60 mg
Transdermal estradiol®–Estraderm®	Prevention/Treatment	0.05 mg patch twice weekly

References [62,63]
1 = intranasal
2 = injection

CONCLUSION

The magnitude of osteoporosis is great among our elderly population. There is now sufficient evidence to support the prevention and treatment of this debilitating disease. Estrogen therapy remains the cornerstone of managing osteoporosis in postmenopausal women and contains beneficial cardiovascular protection properties as well. Supplemental calcium administration is necessary in all patients who are calcium deficient. Although resistance to calcitonin therapy may develop within 24 months of use, it may be advantageous in patients who are experiencing acute fracture pain. Alendronate sodium and raloxifene are promising newer agents for preventing and treating postmenopausal osteoporosis. Because raloxifene has demonstrated positive effects on the skeletal system as well as the cardiovascular system, it may be used as an alternative to patients who cannot tolerate estrogen. As other medications become available, this will provide clinicians with a greater range of pharmacotherapeutic choices for managing this illness. Early recognition of osteoporosis and prompt administration of non-pharmacologic and pharmacologic therapies are extremely important in managing this crippling disease in the postmenopausal population.

REFERENCES

1. Riggs BL, Melton LJ. Involutional osteoporosis. N Engl J Med 1986; 314(26): 1676-86.

2. Osteoporosis. IN: Berg RL, Cassells JS, eds. The second fifty years: promoting health and preventing disability. Washington, DC: National Academy Press, 1990: 76-100.

3. Chisholm MA, Mulloy AL. Management of osteoporosis. Journal of Geriatric Drug Therapy 1996;11(1):5-16.

4. Who are candidates for prevention and treatment for osteoporosis? Osteoporosis Int 1997;7:1-6.

5. Ray NF, Chan JK, Thamer M, Melton LJ. Medical expenditures for the treatment of osteoporotic fractures in the United States in 1995: Report from the National Osteoporosis Foundation. J Bone Miner Res. 1997;12(1):24-35.

6. Melton LJ, Riggs BL. Epidemiology of age-related fractures. In: Avioli LV, ed. The osteoporotic syndrome. New York: Gune & Stralton, 1983; 45-72.

7. Kelsey JF. Osteoporosis: prevalence and incidence. In: Proceedings of the NIH consensus development conference, April 2-4, 1984: 25-8.

8. Cummings SR, Kelsey JL, Nevitt MC, O'Dowd KJ. Epidemiology of osteoporosis and osteoporotic fractures. Epidemiol Rev 1985; 7: 178-208.

9. Cummings SR, Rubin SM, Black D. The future of hip fractures in the United States: numbers, costs, and potential effects of postmenopausal estrogen. Clin Orthopaedics & Related Research 1990; 252: 163-6.

10. Parfitt AM. Bone remodeling: relationship to the amount and the structure of bone, and the pathogenesis and prevention of fractures. In: Riggs BL, Melton LJ, eds. Osteoporosis: etiology, diagnosis, and management. New York: Raven Press, 1988: 45-93.

11. Kleerekoper M, Avioli LV. Evaluation and treatment of postmenopausal osteoporosis. In: Favus MJ, ed. Primer on the Metabolic Bone Diseases and Disorders of Mineral Metabolism, 1st edition. Kelseyville, CA: American Society for Bone and Mineral Research, 1990: 151-154.

12. Mulloy AL, Weinstein RS. Clinical management of osteoporosis. Journal of the Medical Association of Georgia. 1994; 83(4): 227-230.

13. Krolner B, Pors Nielsen S. Bone mineral content of the lumbar spine in normal and osteoporotic women: cross-sectional and longitudinal studies. Clin Sci 1982; 62(3): 329-36.

14. Aloia JF, Vaswani A, Ellis K, Yuen K, Cohn SH. A model for involutional bone loss. J Lab Clin Med 1985; 106(6): 630-7.

15. Riggs BL. Overview of osteoporosis. West J Med 1991; 154(1):63-77.

16. Weinstein RS. Bone involvement in multiple myeloma. Am J Med 1992; 93(6):591-598.

17. Kanis JA, Melton LJ III, Christiansen C, Johnston CC, Khaltaev N. The diagnosis of osteoporosis. J Bone Miner Res 1994;9:1137-41.

18. Melton LJ, Kan SH, Wahner HW, Riggs BL. Lifetime fracture risk: an approach to hip fracture risk assessment based on bone mineral density and age. J Clin Epidemiol 1988; 41(10): 985-94.

19. Cummings SR, Black DM, Nevitt MC, Browner W, Cavley J, Ensrud K, Genant HK, Palermo L, Scott J, Vogt TM. Bone density at various sites for prediction of hip fractures. Lancet 1993; 341: 72-75.

20. Hui SL, Slemenda CW, Johnson CC Jr. Baseline measurement of bone mass predicts fractures in white women. Ann Intern Med 1989; 111(5): 355-361.

21. Riggs BL, Melton LJ. The prevention and treatment of osteoporosis. N Eng J Med 1992; 327(9):620-627.

22. Tosteson AN, Rosenthal DI, Melton LJ, Weinstein MC. Cost effectiveness of screening perimenopausal white women for osteoporosis: bone densitometry and hormone replacement therapy. Ann Intern Med 1990; 113(8): 594-603.

23. Consensus Conference: osteoporosis. JAMA 1984; 242: 799-802.

24. Institute of Medicine, National Research Council. Summary statement on calcium and related nutrients. 1997;S1-S14.

25. Consensus development conference. Diagnosis, prophylaxis and treatment of osteoporosis. Am J Med. 1993;94:646-50.

26. Christiansen C, Riis P. Consensus development conference: prevention and treatment of osteoporosis. Nordisk Medicin 1991; 106(5):145-7.

27. Wild RA. Estrogen: effects on the cardiovascular tree. Obstet Gynecol. 1996;87:27S-35S.

28. Grodsetin F, Stampfer MJ, Manson JE, Colditz GA, Willett WC, Rosner B, Speizer FE, Hennekens CH. Postmenopausal estrogen and progestin use and the risk of cardiovascular disease. N Eng J Med. 1996;335(7);453-61.

29. Hulley SH, Grady D, Bush T, Furberg C, Herrington D, Riggs B, Vittinghoff E. Randomized trial of estrogen plus progestin for secondary prevention of coronary heart disease in postmenopausal women. JAMA. 1998;280:605-613.

30. Ettinger B, Genant HK, Cann CE. Postmenopausal bone loss is prevented by treatment with low-dosage estrogen with calcium. Ann Intern Med 1987; 106(1): 40-5.

31. Riggs BL, Khosla S. Practical clinical management. In: Riggs BL, Melton LJ, Editors. Osteoporosis: Etiology, Diagnosis, and Management, 2nd ed. New York: Lippincott-Raven Publishers, 1995: 487-502.

32. The Writing Group for the PEPI Trial. Effects of hormone therapy on bone mineral densisty: results from the postmenopausal estrogen/progestin interventions (PEPI) trial. JAMA. 1996;276:1389-96.

33. Speroff, L. Postmenapausal hormone therapy and breast cancer. Obstet Gynecol. 1996;87:44S-54S.

34. Bergkvist L, Adami HO, Person I, Bergstrom R, Krusemo UB. Prognosis after breast cancer diagnosis in women exposed to estrogen and estrogen-progestogen replacement therapy. Am J Epidemiol 1989; 130(2): 221-8.

35. Barrett-Connor E, Bush TL. Estrogen and coronary heart disease in women. JAMA 1991; 265(14): 1861-7.

36. Colditz GA, Hankinson SE, Hunter DJ, Willett WC, Manson JE, Stampfer MJ, Hennekens C, Rosner B, Speizer FE. The use of estrogens and progestins and the risk of breast cancer in postmenopause women. N Eng J Med 1995; 332(24): 1589-93.

37. Draper MW, Flowers DE, Huster WJ, Nelid JA, Harper KD, Arnaud C. A controlled trial of raloxifene (LY1 39481) HCL: impact on bone turnover and serum lipid profile in healthy postmenopausal women. J Bone Miner Res 1996;11(6):835-42.

38. Delmas PD, Bjarnason NH, Mitlak BH, Ravoux AC, Shah AS, Huster WJ, Draper M, Christianen C. Effects of raloxifene on bone mineral desnisty, serum cholesterol concentrations, and uterine endometrium in postmenopausal women. N Engl J Med 1997;337(23):1641-7.

39. Ettinger B, Black D, Cummings S, Genant H. Raloxifene reduces the risk of incident vertebral fractures; 24 month interim analysis (abstract). Osteoporosis International 1998;8 (suppl 3);11.

40. Walsh BW, Kuller LH, Wild RA, Paul S, Farmer M, Lawrence JB, Shah AS, Anderson PW. Effects of raloxifene on serum lipids and coagulation factors in healthy postmenapausal women. JAMA. 1998;279(18):1445-51.

41. Wallach S, Farley JR. Baglink DJ, Brenner-Gati L. Effects of calcitonin on bone quality and osteoblastic function. Calcif Tissue Int 1993; 52(5): 335-339.

42. Reginster JY. Effect of calcitonin on bone mass and fracture rates. Am J Med 1991; 91: Suppl 5B; 19S-22S.

43. Thamsborg G, Strom TL, Sykulski R, Brinch E, Nielsen HK, Sorensen OH. Effect of different doses of nasal salmon calcitonin on bone mass. Calcif Tissue Int 1991; 48(5): 302-7.

44. Montemurro L, Schiraldi G, Fraioli P, Tosi G, Riboldi A, Rizzato G. Prevention of glucocorticoid-induced osteoporosis with salmon calcitonin in sarcoid patients. Calcif Tissue Int 1991; 49(2): 71-76.

45. Kleerekoper M, Avioli LV. Evaluation and treatment of postmenopausal osteoporosis. In: Favus, MJ. Primer on the Metabolic bone diseases and disorders of mineral metabolism. New York: Raven Press, 1993; 223-229.

46. Rodan GA, Balena R. Bisphosphonates in the treatment of metabolic bone diseases. Ann Med 1993; 25(4): 373-378.

47. Gertz BJ, Holland SD, Kline WR, Matuszewski BK, Porras AG. Clinical Pharmacology of alendronate sodium. Osteoporosis Int 1993; 3 (Suppl): S13-16.

48. Chestnut CH, McClung MR, Ensrud KE, Bell NH, Genant HK, Harris ST, Singer FR, Stock JL, Yood RA, Delmas PD et al. Alendronate treatment of the postmenopausal osteoporotic woman: effect of multiple dosages on bass mass and bone remolding. Am J Med 1995; 99(2): 144-152.

49. Liberman UA, Weiss SR, Broll J, Minnie HW, Quan H, Bell NH, Rodriguez-Portales J, Downs, RW, Dequeker J, Favus M, Seeman E, Recker RR, Capizzi T, Santora A, Lombardi A, Shah R, Hirsch L, Karpf DB. Effects of oral alendronate on bone mineral density and the incidence of fractures in postmenopausal osteoporosis. N Eng J Med 1995; 333(22): 1437-1443.

50. Chestnut CH, Harris ST. Short-term effect of alendronate on bone mass and bone remodeling in postmenopausal women. Osteoporosis Int 1993; Suppl 3: S17-S19.

51. Adami S, Broni MC, Broggini M, Carratelli L, Carysi I, Laurenzi M, Lombardi A, NorbiatoG, Ortolani S. Treatment of postmenopausal osteoporosis with continuous daily oral alendronate in comparison with either placebo or intranasal salmon calcitonin. Osteoporosis Int 1993; Suppl 3: S21-S27.

52. Karpf DB, Shapiro DR, Seeman E, Ensrud KE, Johnston CC Jr, Adami S, Harris ST, Santora AC2nd, Hirsh LJ, Oppenheimer L, Thompson D. Prevention of nonvertebral fractures by alendronate: a meta-analysis. JAMA. 1997;227(14):1159-64.

53. Black DM, Cummings SR, Karpf DB, Cauley JA, Thompson DE, Nevitt MC, Bauer DC, Genant HK, Haskell WL, Marcus R, Ott SM, Torner JC, Quandt SA, Reiss TF, Ensrud KE. Randomised trial of effect of alendronate on risk of fracture in women with existing vertebral fractures. Lancet. 1996;348:1535-41.

54. Ensrud KE, Black DM, Palermo L, Bauer DC, Barrett-Connor E, Quandt SA, Thompson DE, Karpf DB. Treatment with alendronate prevents fractures in women at highest risk. Arch Intern Med. 1997;157(22):2617-24.

55. Stock JL, Bell NH, Chestnut CH3rd, Ensrud KE, Genant HK, Harris ST, McClung MR, Singer FR, Yood RA, Pryor-Tillotson S, Wei L, Santora AC 2nd. Increments in bone density of the lumbar spine and hip and suppression of bone turnover are maintained after discontinuation of alendronate in postmenopausal women. Am J Med. 1997;103(4):291-7.

56. McClung M, Clemmesen B, Daifotis A, Gilchrist NL, Eisman J, Weinstein RS, Fuleihan Gel H, Reda C, Yates AJ, Ravin P. Alendronate prevents postmenopausal bone loss in women without osteoporosis. A double-blind, randomized, controlled trial. Alendronate Osteoporosis Prevention Study Group. Ann Intern Med 1998;128(4):253-261.

57. Hosking D, Chilvers CE, Christiansen C, Ravn P, Wasnich R, Ross P, McClung M, Balske A, Thompson D, Daley M, Yates AJ. Prevention of bone loss with alendronate in postemenopausal women under 60 years of age. N Engl J Med 1998;338(8):485-92.

58. Eastell R. Treatment of postmenopausal osteoporosis. N Engl J Med 1998; 338(11):736-746.

59. Tinetti ME, Baker DI, McAvay G, Claus EB, Garrett P, Gottschalk M, Koch ML, Trainor K, Horwitz RI. A mutifactorial intervention to reduce the risk of falling among elderly people living in the community. N Engl J Med 1994;331(13):821-7.

60. Felson DR, Zhang Y, Hannan MT, Kiel DP, Wilson PW, Anderson JJ. The effect of postemenapausal estrogen therapy on bone density in elderly women. N Engl J Med, 1993;329(16):1141-6.

61. Sagraves R, Letassy NA. Gynecological Disorders, in Young LY, Koda-Kimble MA (ed): Applied Therapeutics: The Clinical Use of Drugs. Vancouver, WA, Applied Therapeutics, Inc.,1995, pp46.1-46.38.

62. American Hospital Formulary Service 98. Drug Information. McEvory GK, Litvak K, Dewey DR et al. (ed). Bethesda, MD. American Society of Health System Phramacists, Inc., 1998.

63. Drug Facts and Comparisons. Kastrup EK, Hebel SK, Rivard R et al. (ed). St. Louis, MO. Facts and Comparisons. 1998.

Osteoarthritis in the Geriatric Patient

Leisa L. Marshall
Susan W. Miller

SUMMARY. Osteoarthritis is a common chronic condition affecting geriatric patients. It is a disease of cartilage degeneration with secondary changes in the bone, leading to pain, a decrease in functional ability, and even disability in some patients. The goals of management of the geriatric patient are to alleviate symptoms and maintain mobility and functioning. Both nonpharmacological and pharmacological therapy are used.

Pharmacological therapy for osteoarthritis includes capsaicin, acetaminophen, nonsteroidal anti-inflammatory agents, and intraarticular injections. Pharmacological therapy should be initiated cautiously in the geriatric patient, as geriatric patients may be at increased risk of adverse reactions from the medications prescribed compared to a younger patient.

This article reviews current treatment guidelines for geriatric patients with osteoarthritis. Acetaminophen is now recommended as the initial oral agent to be used in the majority of geriatric patients. Topical capsaicin may also provide symptom relief in many patients. Nonsteroidal anti-inflammatory agents are recommended for use if acetaminophen is ineffective, or during periods of inflammation. The patient's concomitant diseases, therapy, and the potential for adverse effects should be carefully considered before a NSAID is recommended. Common adverse effects of the NSAIDs are reviewed. *[Article copies available for a fee from The Haworth Document Delivery Service: 1-800-342-9678. E-mail address: getinfo@haworthpressinc.com <Website: http://www.haworthpressinc.com>]*

Leisa L. Marshall, PharmD, CGP, is Clinical Assistant Professor, and Susan W. Miller, PharmD, FASCP, CGP, is Professor, both at Mercer University Southern School of Pharmacy, Atlanta, GA 30341.

[Haworth co-indexing entry note]: "Osteoarthritis in the Geriatric Patient." Marshall, Leisa L., and Susan W. Miller. Co-published simultaneously in *Journal of Geriatric Drug Therapy* (Pharmaceutical Products Press, an imprint of The Haworth Press, Inc.) Vol. 12, No. 4, 1999, pp. 21-43; and: *Musculoskeletal Drug Therapy for Geriatric Patients* (ed: Marie A. Chisholm, and James W. Cooper) Pharmaceutical Products Press, an imprint of The Haworth Press, Inc., 1999, pp. 21-43. Single or multiple copies of this article are available for a fee from The Haworth Document Delivery Service [1-800-342-9678, 9:00 a.m. - 5:00 p.m. (EST). E-mail address: getinfo@haworthpressinc.com].

KEYWORDS: osteoarthritis, geriatric patients, acetaminophen, capsaicin, nonsteroidal anti-inflammatory drugs, renal impairment

INTRODUCTION

Osteoarthritis is the most common form of arthritis in the United States. It is a major cause of decreased quality of life and disability for geriatric patients.[1-5] Most individuals over the age of 65 have pathologic evidence of osteoarthritis, with about half of these individuals experiencing some symptoms.[4,6-8] Osteoarthritis is a disease of cartilage degeneration with secondary changes in the underlying bone that result in the pain and functional limitations the patient experiences.

Medications are commonly used to decrease the patient's symptoms. Medication therapy is an important component of the medical management of a patient with osteoarthritis, but is only one component. In 1995 the American College of Rheumatology published "Guidelines for the medical management of osteoarthritis: Part I. Osteoarthritis of the hip and Part II. Osteoarthritis of the Knee."[3,9] Other more recent articles have added to their recommendations for the management of osteoarthritis. This article will review the epidemiology, pathophysiology, signs and symptoms, and treatment for osteoarthritis in the geriatric patient.

EPIDEMIOLOGY

Most individuals over the age of 65 have radiographic evidence of osteoarthritis.[1,7,10] The prevalence of osteoarthritis in all joint sites increases with age. Although the majority of geriatric patients may have osteoarthritis, only some experience severe symptoms or disability. The percentage of patients with osteoarthritis categorized as moderate to severe does increase with age, to approximately 30% of the geriatric patients with osteoarthritis of the knee, and 50% of the geriatric patients with osteoarthritis of the hip.[10] Overall, in the United States, osteoarthritis of the knee causes more disability than that of other joints.[1] Osteoarthritis of the knee is also more common than osteoarthritis of the hip.[1]

RISK FACTORS

Obesity as a young adult increases the risk of developing symptomatic ostearthritis of the knee as an older individual, particularly among female patients.[1,4] Strenuous, high intensity exercise or sports activity as a young adult is a controversial risk factor for osteoarthritis.[4] Continued high intensity exercise or sports activity with an injured or abnormal joint is clearly associated with an increased risk of osteoarthritis in the affected joint.[4,10] Repetitive overuse of a joint over many hours of the day, as seen with some vocational activities, also increases the risk of osteoarthritis in the affected joint.[1,11] The role of heredity as a risk factor has been identified with osteoarthritis of the hands, particularly in women.[11] Genetic changes in the collagen and cartilage of affected joints is being studied and may yield useful information in the future.[1,4,11]

PATHOPHYSIOLOGY

The pathology of osteoarthritis is not completely understood but it reflects joint damage and the reaction of the entire joint area to that damage. It is a disease of cartilage deterioration involving not only the cartilage but also the synovium, subchondral bone, ligaments, and nerve innervation in the area.[1] Osteoarthritis may result from excessive stress that exceeds the repair capacity of the tissues of the joint area or insufficient ability of these tissues to repair under normal stress.[1] Early in the disease there is hypertrophic repair of the cartilage with the cartilage appearing thicker than normal.[1] In this stage the cartilage has an increase in water and proteoglycan content. With time there is a decline in water and proteoglycan and a thinning of the cartilage. The cartilage softens and is unable to repair itself sufficiently, leading to a loss of cartilage and the secondary effects of cartilage loss.[1,8,11] The secondary effects of the cartilage deterioration cause the symptoms, since the cartilage itself is not innervated.[4] Bone remodeling and hypertrophy occur. Osteophytes form from the growth of cartilage and bone at the joint margins.[1] This can limit the range of motion of the joint. Joint capsule distention from joint deformity, bony proliferation, pressure in subchondral bone, and damage to ligaments, tendons, and fascia are among the secondary effects that result in the symptoms of the disease.[1,4]

NATURAL HISTORY OF THE OSTEOARTHRITIC PROCESS

The natural course of osteoarthritis is different for each patient and within each patient varies over time.[6] A geriatric patient may have mild or more severe radiographic evidence of osteoarthritis and experience only mild symptoms. In fact, most geriatric individuals have pathologic evidence of osteoarthritis of the knee or hip, with only some of these individuals having symptoms or disability. Other patients experience symptoms, limitations in functional ability, and even disability.[6,7] The disease progresses faster in the joints of the hand than in the knee or hip joint.

SIGNS AND SYMPTOMS

The signs and symptoms a patient experiences depend upon the progression of the disease and the joints affected. Disease onset is usually insidious with joint discomfort in the involved joints.[12] Joint involvement is usually asymmetrical with most patients having minimal systemic symptoms. Joint involvement may become symmetric later in the disease. Early in the disease the patient will complain of pain after joint use that is relieved by rest.[13] As the disease progresses, the pain will occur with rest, as well as with use of the joint. The patient may feel stiffness after inactivity. The joint area becomes enlarged from increased synovial fluid or synovitis, alterations in the cartilage, and the proliferative response of the surrounding bone.[13,14] Other signs of osteoarthritis include crackling on motion, local tenderness, and a variable amount of effusion.[4,15] The patient will have local symptoms, unlike a patient with rheumatoid arthritis who will have systemic manifestations of the disease.

Chronic synovial inflammation, which is a hallmark of rheumatoid arthritis, is often absent in osteoarthritis.[12] This is a key distinction between osteoarthritis and rheumatoid arthritis that makes chronic use of systemic nonsteroidal anti-inflammatory drugs and corticosteroids less than rational. Synovial fluid analysis reveals an increased cell count, but few other abnormalities.[10] There are no specific laboratory tests indicative of osteoarthritis. However, laboratory tests are used to exclude other causes of the symptoms. Serum electrolytes, a complete blood count, and a urinalysis are usually normal unless the geriatric patient has a co-morbid condition affecting these tests. The erythrocyte sedimentation rate is also usually normal. It may be elevated in a patient with erosive inflammatory or generalized osteoarthritis.[13] Progressive changes seen on x-ray include joint space narrowing, subchondral bony sclerosis, and osteophyte and cyst formations at the joint margins.[10]

AFFECTED SITES

The most common sites a geriatric patient may have osteoarthritis are the hand, hip, spine, knee, and foot. In the hand the distal interphalangeal, proximal interphalangeal, and carpometacarpal joints are often affected.[2] Osteoarthritis of the proximal interphalangeal and distal interphalangeal joints may be inflammatory with redness, heat, and tenderness in the area.[16] Bony enlargements at the distal interphalangeal joints are termed Heberden's nodes, while those at the proximal interphalangeal joints are termed Bouchard's nodes.[2] Symptoms usually begin in patients over the age of 55, with women being affected more often than men.[2] There is a strong hereditary component, particularly in women.[2] The appearance of these nodes is usually insidious, developing over several years.[13] A few patients may have an acute onset, accompanied by erythema and swelling.[2,10] A patient over 70 may have Heberden's or Bouchard's nodes that developed when they were younger. The patient will have some limitation in hand function, but no longer complain of the pain and tenderness experienced when the nodes developed twenty years ago.[6] There is also an erosive form of osteoarthritis of the hands that develops in women in their thirties. Within twenty years the hands will exhibit deformities, but the patient will be relatively pain free.[2,11]

Osteoarthritis of the hip is seen in geriatric patients more often than in younger patients. It is usually unilateral.[2] The symptoms develop over time with increasing pain and gait changes. The patient may begin to walk with a limp and have difficulty arising from a seated position.[2] The patient will complain of pain to the groin and anterior or lateral thigh on the side of the affected hip, morning stiffness, range of motion limitations, and pain on motion.[3] Patients may have referred pain in the knee, sciatic area, or buttocks.[13] The pain and functional impairment can cause increasing disability.

Osteoarthritis of the knee is also commonly seen in geriatric patients. The patient typically has morning stiffness with knee pain that worsens with ambulation.[9] Joint motion may be limited with gait changes. The patient may experience "gelling," or localized stiffness of short duration that is relieved by activity.[4] The joint area may be tender to palpation with bony enlargement and muscle atrophy.[9,13] If inflammation is present it is usually mild compared to an affected joint in rheumatoid arthritis.[9]

Osteoarthritis of the spine is less common than osteoarthritis of the hip and knee, but can cause intense pain from compression of nerve routes.[13] The intervertebral discs, vertebral bodies, or posterior apophyseal articulations are involved in osteoarthritis of the spine.[10] Osteoarthritis of the foot commonly affects the first metatarsal phalangeal joint, causing tenderness, swelling and pain.[2] This must be differentiated from gout, where uric acid crystals would be found in the joint.[2]

GOALS OF OSTEOARTHRITIS MANAGEMENT

The goals of management of the geriatric patient with osteoarthritis are to control the pain and maintain mobility and functioning.[3] Therapy should decrease joint stiffening, decrease disability, and maintain or improve the patient's quality of life. However, the pathological process causing the symptoms is irreversible.[17] The joint alterations progress with time in most patients.[17] The patient and their family members should be educated about the disease and therapy for the disease.[3,18] Compliance with therapy should improve the patient's symptoms. Therapeutic options are nonpharmacological therapy, pharmacological therapy, and orthopedic surgery. Nonpharmacological and pharmacological therapy will be emphasized in this review.

When designing a treatment plan the patient's other medical problems, as well as age-related changes in pharmacokinetics and pharmacodynamics should be considered.[6] The medications prescribed for osteoarthritis may worsen a pre-existing condition. If a patient has hypertension, cardiovascular disease, peptic ulcer disease, or renal or hepatic disorders, these conditions would influence the choice of therapy.[3] Changes in body composition with age and the decline in renal function may increase the risk of adverse effects from prescribed medications. Prior adverse reactions to specific medications should also be considered.

NONPHARMACOLOGICAL THERAPY

The role of nonpharmacological therapy in the management of osteoarthritis in a geriatric patient cannot be over-emphasized. Nonpharmacological therapy can reduce pain and increase mobility and function in many patients without the risks of adverse effects or worsening of co-existing conditions possible with pharmacological therapy.[6] Nonpharmacological therapy should begin with patient education. A geriatric patient's life will be greatly affected by osteoarthritis. Patients and their family members should learn about the disease, prognosis, therapeutic alternatives, and realistic outcomes from the therapeutic alternatives.[8] Patients living in the community should be encouraged to participate in programs available in their area for patients with osteoarthritis. The Arthritis Foundation (phone # 1-800-933-7023; web site: http://www.arthritis.org) has numerous educational materials for patients and their family members. Local chapters of the Arthritis Foundation and many hospitals sponsor or offer patient education, self-help, and exercise programs. Patients who have attended self-help courses by the Arthritis Foundation report an improvement in quality of life.[3,6] Patients living in senior retirement communities or assisted living facilities should be made aware of the programs offered by their facility. Physical therapists and occupational therapists often design appropriate exercises and activities for the patient in a long-term care facility.

Other than patient education, nonpharmacological therapy that should be employed includes diet, rest, exercise, occupational therapy, physical therapy, and assistive devices.[3,6,8] Surgical procedures may be necessary and beneficial for a patient with severe symptomatic osteoarthritis who fails to respond to nonpharmacological and pharmacological therapy. Through sensible dietary modification and appropriate aerobic exercise, the patient should loose weight if obese and the weight-bearing joints are those affected. Proper regular exercise will maintain the muscles surrounding the arthritic joint.

Patients may have a consult with a physical therapist for instruction in low impact or no impact exercises, such as swimming or stationary cycle, to strengthen the muscles surrounding the arthritic joint and to increase the range of motion. The physical therapist will evaluate the patient's muscle strength, range of motion, pain, and functional ability.[3] Isotonic or isometric exercises may be used. Contracting the quadriceps muscle while moving the joint against resistance is an example of an isotonic exercise; whereas contracting the quadriceps muscle while seated is an example of an isometric exercise.[12] Quadriceps strengthening exercises and straight leg raises have been shown to improve function and decrease pain in patients with osteoarthritis of the knee.[9,10]

For a patient with osteoarthritis of the hip exercises to strengthen the hip abductors and extensors and maintain range of motion are beneficial.[3] Performing isometric exercises and participating in aerobic aquatic exercise programs are often recommended for their beneficial effects of reducing symptoms and maintaining or improving function.[6,8] A patient should begin an exercise program gradually under professional guidance and be advised to decrease the exercise intensity if severe pain or inflammation develops. If acute inflammation, swelling, or pain is present, the patient should not exercise.[12] Rest is important in relieving pain after activity or in weight-bearing joints. Short periods of rest are beneficial, but long periods of immobility may eventually worsen the condition.[8] The physical therapist may recommend heat therapy to alleviate the pain, especially just prior to exercise. Heat therapy is beneficial for most patients. Examples of heat therapy include warm baths or showers or the cautious use of moist heat packs.[12] Alternatively, cold has been helpful in pain relief in some patients.[19]

An occupational therapist will evaluate the patient's environment and ability to perform activities of daily living. The occupational therapist will then recommend environmental changes and assistive devices, for example, chairs of appropriate seat height or raised toilet seats, to increase the independence of the patient. For patients with osteoarthritis of the hip or knee, the physician and physical therapist may recommend the use of a cane or walker to reduce the force on the weight-bearing joint to allow for decreased pain on ambulating. Aerobic aquatic exercise programs have been shown to have a positive effect on the patient's aerobic conditioning, improve muscle strength and functional ability, and reduce pain.[3,4,15] The Arthritis Foundation has developed and sponsors an aerobic aquatic program, consisting of water exercises, that does not require the ability to swim.

PHARMACOLOGICAL THERAPY

Treatment Guidelines

If nonpharmacological therapy fails to provide adequate relief, pharmacological therapy will be needed. The patient should understand that they should continue to use the nonpharmacological therapy as directed by the physician, even when over-the-counter or prescription medications have been prescribed. Pharmacological therapy should be initiated cautiously in the geriatric patient. The physiologic changes with aging, concurrent disease states, and medications for these disease states places the geriatric patient at increased risk of adverse reactions from the medications prescribed for osteoarthritis.[6]

As mentioned earlier, the American College of Rheumatology recently published "Guidelines for the Medical Management of Osteoarthritis: Part I. Osteoarthritis of the Hip and Part II. Osteoarthritis of the Knee."[3,9] These guidelines discuss the medical management of patients with osteoarthritis of the hip and knee in detail. For patients for whom nonpharmacological modalities are inadequate, they recommend acetaminophen as the initial medication of choice for systemic treatment.[3,9] This recommendation was based on usual symptomatology, and a comparison of the efficacy, safety, and cost of acetaminophen versus full-dose nonsteroidal anti-inflammatory drugs (NSAIDs).[3,9]

For many years NSAIDs were prescribed initially for their analgesic and anti-inflammatory properties. The adverse effect profile of the NSAIDs is the primary reason for not recommending them as initial agents in osteoarthritis.[3,9] Since geriatric patients experience a higher incidence of adverse effects from NSAIDs than younger patients, a trial of acetaminophen as the initial oral agent is even more imperative in this population.[6,14,20] Although inflammation may be present intermittently in osteoarthritis, analgesics appear to be effective for sources of pain in osteoarthritis other than the inflammation.[4] Several studies have shown acetaminophen to be just as effective as NSAIDs in improving outcomes for patients with osteoarthritis.[20,22]

The topical analgesic capsaicin cream is also recommended as appropriate for monotherapy or adjunctive therapy for osteoarthritis of the knee or other affected joints.[9,10] If a patient's response is inadequate to acetaminophen or capsaicin cream, a low dose of ibuprofen or a non-acetylated salicylate should be tried.[3,9] Ibuprofen is recommended for use on an as needed basis at a dose of less than 1600mg per day.[3,9] A patient's symptoms will differ slightly each day, so an inexpensive agent with a relatively short half life and lower incidence of side-effects at low doses is a reasonable suggestion.[3,9] Many patients may need to take scheduled ibuprofen, at doses up to 400mg qid for relief of symptoms.[3,9] Alternatively, a non-acetylated salicylate could be used if a patient does not have adequate relief from nonpharmacological therapy, acetaminophen, and topical capsaicin.[3,9] Nonacetylated salicylates have a lower incidence of gastric and renal toxicity than full-dose nonsteroidal anti-inflammatory medications.[3,9,15]

If a patient does not respond adequately to a nonacetylated salicylate or a low dose of a NSAID such as ibuprofen, a full dose NSAID may be needed.[3,9] Since the inflammation of osteoarthritis may be intermittent, regular use of NSAIDs could be limited to periods when more conservative measures are inadequate.[6,14] Patient response to particular NSAIDs is highly variable which may necessitate trials with several different agents. The advantages and disadvantages of particular NSAIDs in the geriatric patient will be discussed later in the section on NSAIDs.

Patients with osteoarthritis of the knee and hands may benefit from occasional steroid injections into the affected joint, but frequent injections should be avoided, as discussed in the section on corticosteroids.[9,13] Oral or parenteral corticosteroid therapy is not indicated for osteoarthritis.[13] Patients with severe osteoarthritis of the hip or knee who have intolerable pain and limitation of function may require surgery.[2] Total joint arthroplasty of the hip and knee is highly successful for most patients in producing pain relief and increasing functional status.[2,3,9]

Medication Therapy

Capsaicin

Capsaicin is a topical analgesic that is effective in relieving the pain of osteoarthritic joints. For example, it is available as a 0.025% and 0.075% cream over-the-counter. Topical capsaicin should be considered for use early in therapy in geriatric patients since it is effective for many patients and does not have systemic side-effects.[9] Geriatric patients respond favorably to topical therapy as many have used topical home remedies for osteoarthritis or other conditions. Capsaicin may be used as monotherapy or in combination with oral agents.[6,9] The patient should gently apply the product to the affected joint(s) two to four times a day.[10] Once the full effect is seen after two to three weeks of continuous use, the patient may be able to decrease the applications to two to three times a day.[10] Patients should be counseled that capsaicin may initially worsen their pain, but this is part of the therapeutic effect. A local anesthetic preparation, e.g., benzocaine, may be used as needed to ameliorate this transitional increase in pain.

The continuous use of topical capsaicin depletes substance P, an endogenous pain producing neuropeptide found in elevated quantities in the synovial fluid of patients with arthritis.[6] Substance P is a mediator of pain impulses from the periphery to the central nervous system.[22] If a patient using capsaicin as monotherapy does not experience adequate symptom relief after several weeks of continuous use, oral analgesic therapy should be recommended.

A geriatric patient may experience adequate symptom relief with topical capsaicin and oral acetaminophen. If not, the continuous use of capsaicin may allow a patient to experience adequate symptom relief with a lower dose of a NSAID than without capsaicin. Capsaicin has the advantage of causing no systemic adverse effects. The only adverse effect commonly experienced is a local stinging or burning upon application, but this does not usually lead to discontinuation of capsaicin.[9] The geriatric patient, or nurse applying the product, should be counseled to wash their hands after applying the product, and to avoid contact with the ocular area. The patient should realize that they must use the product continuously, at least three times a day, for it to be effective.[22]

Acetaminophen

Acetaminophen should be recommended as the initial oral agent for the majority of geriatric patients with osteoarthritis, to be used in conjunction with nonpharmacological therapies.[3,4,9,12,15,23] Acetaminophen is an analgesic agent that does not have anti-inflammatory effects. Acetaminophen is inexpensive, causes relatively fewer adverse effects than the nonsteroidal anti-inflammatory drugs (NSAIDs), has the potential for fewer drug-drug interactions, and provides relief through analgesia for some patients with osteoarthritis.[3,4,9,20] As mentioned above, concerns about the role of inflammation in causing the pain of osteoarthritis in some patients, studies comparing the efficacy of acetaminophen versus ibuprofen, and an increased recognition of the adverse effects of chronic NSAID use lead to the current recommendations.[3,4,9,20,21] Acetaminophen does not commonly cause the gastrointestinal adverse effects that are often associated with NSAIDs.[6,23] It also has a lower incidence of renal adverse effects, but can cause tubular necrosis.[24] Acetaminophen has no effect on platelet aggregation or bleeding time. A recent study did find acetaminophen use to be among factors associated with an increased risk for international normalized ratios higher than desired in patients taking warfarin.[25] However, the study was conducted by interview. Further study of how and if acetaminophen potentiates warfarin's anti-coagulant effect would be needed to alter recommendations for acetaminophen use.[25]

The patient may take acetaminophen on an as needed basis prior to activities that usually cause pain. They may benefit from prophylactic acetaminophen prior to the morning routine of arising and dressing, or prior to exercise. During periods of pain acetaminophen will need to be used on a scheduled basis.[6] The dosage used should be monitored closely to avoid the development of hepatotoxicity. Acetaminophen does have the disadvantage of being more hepatotoxic than the NSAIDs approved for osteoarthritis. Dosages of three to four grams a day for a year have resulted in liver damage.[22,23] A geriatric patient with a previous history of liver disease, who ingests alcohol regularly, or who fasts, is at increased risk of hepatotoxicity from acetaminophen, and should avoid taking acetaminophen on a regular basis.[6,23]

A geriatric patient with no prior history of suspected or documented liver damage may take 500mg to 650mg every six hours on an as needed, or scheduled, basis.[3,9,10] Chronic doses of up to 4000mg per day have been used, but the patient would be at increased risk of hepatotoxicity.[3,9,23] For a patient with a creatinine clearance of less than 10ml/minute, caution is warranted as the metabolites will accumulate, causing toxicity.[22] Liver enzymes tests and liver function tests should be monitored in patients taking acetaminophen chronically. There is little data in geriatric patients regarding the chronic use of acetaminophen with other hepatotoxic agents, such as valproate, isoniazid, pyrizinamide, troglitazone, or the HMG-CoA reductase inhibitors. The older patient may be at increased risk of liver damage with concurrent use of these agents.

Nonsteroidal Anti-Inflammatory Drugs: Nonacetylated Salicylates and Aspirin

Some patients will not have adequate relief from acetaminophen, and will experience much greater relief of symptoms by taking a nonacetylated salicylate or aspirin. Table 1 contains the usual dosage range for geriatric patients for aspirin and several nonacetylated salicylates.[22,26,27] Aspirin could be used on an as needed or scheduled basis for analgesic and anti-inflammatory effects. Aspirin has analgesic effects at low to moderate doses but requires more than 3.6 grams per day for anti-inflammatory effects.[10] If a patient were being monitored for anti-inflammatory effects, serum salicylate concentrations would need to be checked, but this is not commonly done in osteoarthritis.[10] In younger patients salicylate concentrations of 15-30mg/dl correlate with anti-inflammatory effects, and concentrations greater than 30mg/dl with toxic effects.[10,28] An elderly patient may experience toxic effects at lower concentrations.[10,29] Aspirin is not often recommended for scheduled chronic use at multiple daily doses because of the high incidence of gastrointestinal distress, gastrointestinal blood loss and the irreversible platelet aggregation associated with the use of aspirin.[3,10,23] Irreversible platelet aggregation occurs with a single dose of aspirin for the life of the platelet, which is seven to ten days. With chronic ingestion of moderate doses, a few patients may even experience acute hemorrhagic gastritis with the passage of large amounts of blood in the stool or the vomiting of blood.

Enteric coated aspirin at low to moderate doses may be an appropriate inexpensive choice for some patients.[8] Enteric coated aspirin causes less gastric mucosal injury than plain or buffered aspirin, but retains anti-inflammatory properties and effects on platelet aggregation.[23] If a patient is scheduled for surgery, aspirin should be discontinued up to one week prior to the surgery, depending on the situation.[23] A patient taking aspirin on a routine basis may be at risk of salicylate toxicity. Symptoms of salicylate toxicity include tinnitus, dizziness, disturbances in balance, nausea and vomiting, agitation, and confusion.[23] Tinnitus may not be a reliable symptom of toxicity in geriatric patients due to functional hearing loss and prior damage to the eighth cranial nerve. An onset of dizziness or balance problems could be used as an indication of salicylate toxicity. Salicylate elimination may be decreased in some patients over age 70, especially those with low serum albumin.[29] Aspirin may also adversely effect renal function and may also cause an elevation in serum transaminase levels.

If a patient with osteoarthritis does not experience adequate control of symptoms with topical capsaicin and acetaminophen, a nonacetylated salicylate (NAS) used on an as needed basis may provide symptom relief. NAS provide analgesia and are anti-inflammatory. A geriatric patient should have decreased pain, stiffness, and swelling after

TABLE 1. Nonsteroidal Anti-Inflammatory Drugs for Osteoarthritis

Medication	Usual dosage range for geriatric patients* (dosage adjustments with decreased creatinine clearance and other considerations)**
Aspirin	2.4-3.6gm/day in divided doses (avoid use in severe renal impairment)
Choline magnesium salicylate	500mg-1gm 1-3 times/day (avoid use in severe renal impairment)
Diflunisal	500mg 2 times/day (CrCl < 50ml/min: decrease dose by 50%; avoid use in severe renal impairment)
Salsalate	500mg-750mg 2-3 times/day (decrease dose with decreased CrCl)
Diclofenac	50mg 3 times/day; 75mg 2 times/day; extended release 100mg/day (decrease dose in patients at increased risk of ADRs: low weight, concomitant meds/diseases)
Etodolac	200mg 3-4 times/day; 300mg 2-4 times/day (for long-term adm a total daily dose of 600mg/day may be used; for patients < 60kg NMT 20mg/kg)
Fenoprofen	300mg-600mg 3-4 times/day (avoid use in moderate/severe renal impairment)
Flurbiprofen	50mg 4 times/day to 100mg 3 times/day (avoid use in moderate/severe renal impairment)
Ibuprofen	200mg-800mg 3-4 times/day (avoid use in moderate/severe renal impairment)
Indomethacin	25mg-3 times/day; 50mg 2 times/day; SR 75mg 1 time/day (avoid use in moderate/severe renal impairment)
Ketoprofen	25mg-50mg 3-4 times/day (NMT 100-15mg/day in patients with mild/moderate renal impairment; avoid use in moderate/severe renal impairment)
Meclofenamate	50mg 3-4 times/day to 100mg 3 times/day (avoid use in moderate/severe renal impairment)
Nabumetone	500mg-750mg 1-2 times/day (dosage adjustment usually not necessary with decreased CrCl, but avoid use in moderate/severe renal impairment)
Naproxen	250mg-500mg 2 times/day (decrease dose in patients with decreased creatinine clearance; avoid use in moderate/severe renal impairment)
Oxaprozin	600mg-1200mg 1 time/day (avoid use in moderate/severe renal impairment)
Sulindac	150mg 2 times/day (avoid use in moderate/severe renal impairment)
Tolmetin	200mg-400mg 3 times/day (avoid use in moderate/severe renal impairment)

*   geriatric patients are at risk of adverse effects even with the usual dosages
**   NSAIDs may further decrease renal function in patients with declining creatinine clearance
Sources: (22,26,27)

taking a NAS. When symptoms are not adequately relieved with as needed administration, a NAS could be used on a scheduled basis. NAS may cause less gastrointestinal distress, bleeding, and renal toxicity than aspirin or the acetic acid, propionic acid, fenamate, pyrazole, or oxicam NSAIDs.[10,15] NAS also do not decrease platelet aggregation. For these reasons NAS are preferred by some physicians and patients.[15] They still cause salicylate toxicity at high serum levels. Serum salicylate levels would need to be monitored if a patient took 3000mg or greater of a NAS daily.[10] Renal function should be monitored when a patient takes a NAS on a regular basis, although they have less adverse effects on the kidney than other NSAIDs. The geriatric patient on salicylate therapy should avoid medications that delay salicylate excretion, for example probenecid, and medications that acidify urine pH, for example, greater than 4gm per day of ascorbic acid. Conversely, medications that alkalinize the urine may cause a decrease in serum salicylate. Examples of medications that alkalinize the urine include antacids, sucralfate, and carbonic anhydrase inhibitors.

Nonsteroidal Anti-Inflammatory Drugs: Acetic Acids, Propionic Acids, Fenamates, Pyrazoles, and Oxicams

A NSAID of the acetic acid, propionic acid, fenamate, pyrazole, or oxicam class may be indicated if joint symptoms are not controlled with nonpharmacological therapy and topical or oral analgesics.[3,4,9] Table 1 contains the usual dosage range for geriatric patients for commonly used NSAIDs.[22,26,27] Table 1 also contains dosage reduction recommendations if the patient has a mildly decreased creatinine clearance. However, most references caution to avoid use of most NSAIDs in patients with moderate to severe renal impairment.[22,26,27] The NSAID will alleviate symptoms in many patients, but will not alter the course of the disease. The patient's other medical problems and therapy must be carefully considered before a NSAID of these classes is recommended. Low dose ibuprofen (< 1600mg/day) on an as needed basis should be tried first, according to the American College of Rheumatology, as mentioned earlier.[3,9] Low dose, as needed, ibuprofen is associated with less gastrointestinal toxicity than scheduled full dose NSAIDs.[3,9]

When response is inadequate to as needed administration of a NSAID, a scheduled NSAID may be prescribed.[2,3,9] NSAIDs are relatively equal in efficacy, but patient response is highly variable to particular NSAIDs.[2,10,30] Patients have even been categorized as "responders" and "nonresponders" to a particular NSAID.[30] If a patient does not respond to one NSAID after a trial of four to six weeks, a different NSAID should be tried. Table 1 contains a list of NSAIDs commonly used for osteoarthritis with suggested doses for the geriatric patient.[22,26,27]

NSAIDs are not recommended as first line therapy for a geriatric patient primarily because of the adverse effects associated with their use. Table 2 summarizes the potential adverse effects, and the increased risk factors for these adverse effects.[6,16,31,32] NSAIDs may cause gastrointestinal, renal, central nervous system, hematological, and hepatic toxicity. The geriatric patient is at increased risk of these adverse effects compared to a younger patient, even at the dosages recommended for the geriatric patient.[16] NSAIDs may also cause hypersensitivity reactions with urticaria or bronchospams.[32]

NSAIDs inhibit the conversion of arachidonic acid to intermediate and terminal prostaglandins, which are proinflammatory and work with other pain producing mechanisms. Cyclooxygenase is the specific converting enzyme which converts arachidonic acid to prostaglandins.[31] The difference between individual NSAID's effects on two isoenzymes of cyclooxygenase, cox-1 and cox-2 are being studied. Cox-1 maintains the normal function of tissues of the body, including the kidney and gastrointestinal tract. Cox-2 is in normal tissues in small quantities, but appears to produce prostaglandins in inflammation and mitogenesis.[31] Therefore, a NSAID that inhibited cox-2 with little or no effect on cox-1 would be effective for inflammation with fewer side-effects.[33] Unfortunately, the majority of the NSAIDs on the market at present preferentially inhibit cox-1. Also, to inhibit cox-2 with no effect on cox-1, a NSAID would need to be approximately 100 times more active against cox-2.[33] Equipotent inhibitors of cox-1 and cox-2 include the active metabolite of nabumetone and etodolac.[33] However, at the concentrations needed to inhibit cox-2 these also inhibit cox-1. Piroxicam, indomethacin, and sulindac are believed to preferentially inhibit cox-1 compared to cox-2.[31] Studies are being conducted on preferential inhibitors of cox-2.

The most common adverse effects observed with the NSAIDs are gastrointestinal. Geriatric patients have a higher incidence of gastrointestinal complications from NSAID use than younger patients.[6,32] Geriatric patients may present with bleeding and gastric ulceration

TABLE 2. Potential Adverse Reactions and Risk Factors for Adverse Reactions to Nonsteroidal Anti-Inflammatory Drugs

Site of potential adverse reaction	Risk factors
Gastrointestinal tract	
Nausea and vomiting	Use of more than one NSAID
Mucosal irritation and erosions	History of peptic ulcer disease
Peptic ulcer disease (gastric ulcers)	Concomitant illness
Gastrointestinal hemorrhage	Increased age
Kidney	
Interference with renal blood flow and glomerular filtration	High renal clearance of an active metabolite of the parent compound
Renal failure (reversible)	Declining creatinine clearance
Tubular function alterations	Congestive heart failure, hypertension, increased age
Increase in serum creatinine; sodium and water retention	Renal artery stenosis, renal disease
Hematologic	
Decreased platelet aggregation (reversible with non-aspirin NSAIDs)	Trauma, surgery
Anemia	Increased age
Central nervous system	
Confusion, headaches, depression	Other medications affecting the CNS
Liver	
Elevated liver enzymes (common), severe hepatotoxicity (less common)	History of hepatitis, alcoholism, congestive heart failure
Allergic reactions	
Asthma, urticaria, photosensitivity	Asthma, aspirin allergy

Sources: (6,16,31,32)

with little warning symptoms.[16,32] Etodolac, diclofenac, ibuprofen, and nabumetone may cause less gastrointestinal toxicity than indomethacin, sulindac, and piroxicam.[6,31,34] NSAIDs should be taken with food or milk to decrease the local damage to the gastric mucosa. The exceptions are the enteric-coated products that should not be taken with milk or antacids.

Most ulcers caused by NSAIDs are gastric ulcers.[31] Duodenal ulcers are most often caused by *Helicobacter pylori*, but NSAIDs are implicated in causing some duodenal ulcers. Misoprostol is the FDA approved agent for the prevention of NSAID induced gastric and duodenal ulcers.[3,10,34] It may be considered in patients at increased risk of NSAID induced ulcers, but the cost-effectiveness of treating osteoarthritis patients on chronic NSAIDs with misoprostol is controversial.[3] Misoprostol also causes unacceptable diarrhea in some patients.[16] Women who still have their uterus may experience spotting due to the uterine contractions caused by misoprostol. The proton-pump inhibitors and histamine 2 receptor antagonists have also been used for the prevention of NSAID induced ulcers.[6,34,35] A recent study comparing misoprostol and the proton-pump inhibitor omeprazole as maintenance therapy for patients on chronic NSAIDs, with recently healed gastric or duodenal ulcers, found that therapy with omeprazole maintained more patients in remission than therapy with misoprostol (61% versus 48%).[36] A similar study comparing ranitidine and omeprazole as maintenance therapy for patients on chronic NSAIDs, with recently healed gastric or doudenal ulcers, found that omeprazole maintained more patients in remission than ranitidine (72% versus 59%).[37]

Patients at increased risk of developing NSAID induced peptic ulcers include all geriatric patients, especially those over 75 years of age. Geriatric patients with a prior history of peptic ulcer disease or gastrointestinal bleeding, patients taking higher doses or chronic doses of NSAIDs, and patients taking other medications that increase the risk of ulcers or bleeding, for example, corticosteroids and warfarin, are at an even greater risk of developing serious gastrointestinal complications and should be considered for ulcer prophylaxis.[3,6,31,38] Misoprostol may be prescribed, or if misoprostol is not appropriate therapy for a patient, a proton-pump inhibitor or an histamine-2 receptor antagonist may be prescribed, even though the proton-pump inhibitor and histamine-2 receptor antagonist are not FDA approved for prophylaxis.[6,35] A product containing a combination of misoprostol and the NSAID diclofenac was released recently. Monthly or bimonthly monitoring of hemoglobin and hematocrit may allow for early detection of NSAID induced gastropathy and decrease NSAID related hospitalization. The therapeutic substitution of acetaminophen for NSAIDs has been shown to decrease NSAID induced hospitalizations from gastropathy in long-term care facility patients.[39]

NSAIDs may also cause renal insufficiency and usually should not be prescribed in patients with declining renal function.[16] If used, a low initial dose should be prescribed. A practical method for determining possible renal effects of NSAIDs in the older adult is to have the patient weigh daily for the first month of usage. Any weight gain of five or more pounds may indicate possible renally-mediated fluid retention. Also, the health care professional should pay careful attention to the patient's renal function by monitoring the serum creatinine and blood urea nitrogen, and estimating the patient's creatinine clearance. Creatinine clearance may be estimated using the Cockroft-Gault formula listed below.[40]

For males Creatinine clearance (CrCl) equals:

$$\{ (140 - \text{patient's age in years}) \times \text{body weight in kg}\} / \{72 \times \text{Ser. Creatinine in mg/dL}\}$$

For females CrCl equals:

$$0.85 \times \text{CrCl determined using formula for males}$$

Patients with hypertension, congestive heart failure, diabetes, hepatic insufficiency, or who are also taking diuretics are at an even increased risk of developing renal adverse effects.[2,3,16] Adverse effects include sodium and water retention, hyperkalemia, increases in serum creatinine and blood urea nitrogen, interstitial nephritis and proteinuria, and renal failure.

Chronic NSAID use over several weeks is also associated with an increase in blood pressure in geriatric patients.[41] A greater increase has been seen in patients already taking antihypertensive medications, but is also seen in patients not taking antihypertensives.[41] A study evaluating the risk of beginning antihypertensive agents in geriatric patients taking NSAIDs found a 1.7 fold increased risk of beginning antihypertensive agents compared to geriatric patients not taking NSAIDs, after potential confounders were considered.[42]

The central nervous system, hepatic, hematological, and hypersensitivity adverse reactions are summarized in Table 2, with increased risk factors listed.[6,16,31,32] Considering the adverse effects associated with NSAIDs, a complete blood count, urinalysis, serum creatinine, blood urea nitrogen, and liver enzyme analysis are recommend prior to prescribing a NSAID for a geriatric patient.[2,16] These laboratory indices should be monitored every one to three months the first six months of therapy, and at least every six months after that, depending upon the patient.[2,16]

Intraarticular Injections

Intraarticular injections of a corticosteroid, sodium hyaluronate, or Hylan G-F 20® may be used for patients with osteoarthritis of the knee. If a patient has effusion, signs of inflammation, and significant joint pain in the knee, aspiration of the fluid and intraarticular injection of a corticosteroid should be considered.[9] Injection of a corticosteroid in a joint should not be performed more than three or four times in a twelve month period in a weight-bearing joint, as more frequent injections may cause cartilage damage.[9,13] They should be reserved for periods of acute joint flare.[13] Intraarticular hip joint injections of a corticosteroid have been useful in some patients when surgery is contraindicated.[3] Oral steroids are not indicated for osteoarthritis.

Sodium hyaluronate and Hylan G-F 20® are two relatively new products indicated for treatment of pain in osteoarthritis of the knee when patients have not had adequate response to nonpharmacological therapy and acetaminophen.[43,44] Hyaluronic acid is a component of synovial fluid that lubricates the joints and helps maintain cartilage function.[6] Hyaluronic acid is reduced in the osteoarthritic joint. Intraarticular injections of sodium hyaluronate or Hylan G-F 20® into osteoarthritic knee joints have been shown to reduce pain in some patients.[43,44]

Alternative Medicine

Glucosamine and chondroitin sulfate are two dietary supplements that have been studied for pain relief in patients with osteoarthritis. Several studies published using injectable and oral forms of these agents are summarized in a recent review.[45] The currently available studies contained study design flaws, and at the present time the Arthritis Foundation does not recommend the use of glucosamine or chondroitin sulfate for osteoarthritis.[45] Glucosamine was well tolerated in the trials, but there was concern with the possibility of bleeding with chondroitin sulfate.[45] A patient asking about using these supplements should be told to consult with their physician, and not to discontinue other therapy. Many patients have reported benefits from oral glucosamine.[45] Chondroitin sulfate should be used with caution in patients with bleeding disorders or on anticoagulant therapy.[45] Patients taking NSAIDs or oral corticosteroids would want to consult with their physician prior to taking chondroitin, as they are already at increased risk of developing gastrointestinal bleeding.

CONCLUSION

The geriatric patient who develops pain and functional limitations from osteoarthritis should first try nonpharmacological therapy to alleviate these symptoms. However, the majority of patients will require pharmacological therapy with one or more agents. Therapy selection and monitoring is imperative to insure that the geriatric patient receives the most appropriate therapy without experiencing significant adverse effects.

REFERENCES

1. Brandt K, Slemenda C. Osteoarthritis: epidemiology, pathology, and pathogenesis. In: Schumacher H, ed. *Primer on the Rheumatic Diseases*. 10th ed. Atlanta, Georgia: Arthritis Foundation; 1993:184-188.

2. Harris C. Osteoarthritis: how to diagnose and treat the painful joint. *Geriatrics*. 1993;48(8):39-46.

3. Hochberg M, Altman R, Brandt K et al. Guidelines for the medical management of osteoarthritis: Part I. Osteoarthritis of the Hip. *Arthritis and Rheumatism*. 1995;38(11):1535-1540.

4. Oddis C. New perspectives on osteoarthitis. *The American Journal of Medicine*. 1996;100(2A):10S-15S.

5. Towheed T, Hochberg M. A systematic review of randomized controlled trials of pharmacologic therapy in osteoarthritis of the hip. *Journal of Rheumatology*. 1997;24(2):349-357.

6. Bagge E, Brooks P. Osteoarthritis in older patients. *Drugs and Aging*. 1995;7(3):176-183.

7. Sharma L, Felson D. Studying how osteoarthritis causes disability: nothing is simple. *Journal of Rheumatology*. 1998;25(1):1-4.

8. Dahl S. Osteoarthritis in the elderly: overview and management. *Clinical Pharmacy Newswatch*. 1996;3(9):1-6.

9. Hochberg M, Altman R, Brandt K et al. Guidelines for the Medical Management of Osteoarhtritis: Part II. Osteoarthritis of the Knee. *Arthritis and Rheumatism*. 1995;38(11):1541-1545.

10. Boh L. Osteoarthritis. In: Joseph T. DiPiro RLT et al., ed. *Pharmacotherapy: a pathophysiologic approach*. third ed. Stamford: Appleton and Lange; 1997:1735-1753.

11. Fife R. Osteoarthritis. In: William R. Hazzard ELB, John P. Blass, ed. *Principles of geriatric medicine and gerontology*. third ed. New York: McGraw-Hill, Inc.; 1994:981-986.

12. Ross C. A comparison of osteoarthritis and rheumatoid arthritis: diagnosis and treatment. *Nurse Practitioner*. 1997;22(9):20-39.

13. Moskowitz R, Goldberg V. Osteoarthritis: clinical features and diagnosis. In: Schumacher H, ed. *Primer on the Rheumatic Diseases*. 10th ed. Atlanta, Georgia: Arthritis Foundation; 1993:188-190.

14. Skeith K, Brocks D. Pharmacokinetic optimisation of the treatment of osteoarthritis. *Clinical Pharmacokinetics.* 1994;26(3):233-242.

15. Dearborn J, Jergesen H. The evaluation and initial management of arthritis. *Primary Care.* 1996;23(2):215-240.

16. Nesher G, Moore T. Clinical presentation and treatment of arthritis in the aged. In: Perry H, ed. *Clinics in geriatric medicine: the aging skeleton.* Vol. 10. Philadelphia: WB Saunders; 1994:659-675.

17. Anderson R. Osteoarthritis. In: Carlson K, Eisenstat S, eds. *Primary Care of Women.* St. Louis: Mosby; 1995:167-172.

18. Blackburn W. Management of osteoarthritis and rheumatoid arthritis: prospects and possibilities. *American Journal of Medicine.* 1996;100(supplement 2A):24S-30S.

19. Oosterveld F, Rasker J. Treating arthritis with locally applied heat or cold. *Semin Arthritis Rheum.* 1994;24:82-90.

20. Bradley J, Brandt K, Katz B et al. Comparison of an antiinflammatory dose of ibuprofen, an analgesic dose of ibuprofen, and acetaminophen in the treatment of patients with osteoarthritis of the knee. *New England Journal of Medicine.* 1991;325:87-91.

21. Bradley J, Brandt K, Katz B et al. Treatment of knee osteoarthritis: relationship of clinical features of joint inflammation to the response to a nonsteroidal antiinflammatory drug or pure analgesic. *J Rheumatol.* 1992;19:1950-1954.

22. Semla T, Beizer J, Higbee M, eds. *Geriatric Dosage Handbook.* 3rd ed. Hudson, Ohio: Lexi-Comp; 1997.

23. Lipman A. Internal Analgesic and Antipyretic Products. In: Covington TR, ed. *Handbook of nonprescription drugs.* Washington: American Pharmaceutical Association; 1996:45-74.

24. Anon. Acetaminophen. In: Threlkeld D, Hagemann R, Brantley A et al., eds. *Drug Facts and Comparisons.* St. Louis, MO: Facts and Comparisons; 1997:247-247f.

25. Hylek E et al. Acetaminophen and other risk factors for excessive warfarin anticoagulation. *Journal of the American Medical Association.* 1998;279:657-672.

26. Threlkeld D, Brantley A, Golshahr V et al., eds. *Drug Facts and Comparisons.* St. Louis, Missouri: Facts and Comparisons; 1997.

27. Lacy C et al., eds. *Drug Information Handbook.* 4th ed. Hudson: Lexi-Comp, Inc.; 1996.

28. Paulus H, Bulpitt K. Nonsteroidal antiinflammatory agents and corticosteroids. In: Schumacher H, Klippel J, Koopmen W, eds. *Primer on the Rheumatic Diseases.* Atlanta: Arthritis Foundation; 1993:298-303.

29. Netter P, Faure G, Regent M et al. Salicylate kinetics in old age. *Clin Pharmacol Ther.* 1985;38:6-11.

30. Walker J, Sheather-Reid R, Carmody J et al. Nonsteroidal antiinflammatory drugs in rheumatoid arthritis and osteoarthritis: support for the concept of "responders and nonresponders." *Arthritis and Rheumatism.* 1997;40(11):1944-1954.

31. Polisson R. Nonsteroidal anti-inflammatory drugs: practical and theoretical considerations in their selection. *The American Journal of Medicine.* 1996;100(2A):31S-36S.

32. Amadio P, Cummings D, Amadio P. Nonsteroidal anti-inflammatory drugs: tailoring therapy to achieve results and avoid toxicity. *Postgraduate Medicine.* 1993;93(4):73-97.

33. deBrum-Fernandes A. New perspectives for nonsteroidal antiinflammatory therapy. *Journal of Rheumatology.* 1997;24(2):246-248.

34. Bjorkman D. Nonsteroidal anti-inflammatory drug-induced gastrointestinal injury. *American Journal of Medicine.* 1996;101(supplement 1A):25S-32S.

35. Hawker G. Prescribing Nonsteroidal antiinflammatory drugs-what's new? *Journal of Rheumatology.* 1997;24(2):243-245.

36. Hawkey C, Karrasch J et al. Omeprazole compared with misoprostol for ulcers associated with nonsteroidal antiinflammatory drugs. *New England Journal of Medicine.* 1998;338(11):727-734.

37. Yeomans N, Tulassy Z et al. A comparison of omeprazole wtih ranitidine for ulcers associated with nonsteroidal antiinflammatory drugs. *New England Journal of Medicine.* 1998;338(11):719-726.

38. Fries J, Williams C, Bloch D et al. Nonsteroidal anti-inflammatory drug-associated gastropathy: incidence and risk factor models. *American Journal of Medicine.* 1991;91:213-222.

39. Cooper J. Consultant pharmacist effect on NSAID costs and gastropathy over a 5-year period. *Consultant Pharmacist.* 1997;12(7):792-796.

40. Cockroft D, Gault M. Prediction of creatine clearance from serum creatinine. *Nephron.* 1976;16:31-41.

41. Johnson A. NSAIDs and blood pressure. *Drugs and Aging.* 1998;12(1):17-27.

42. Gurwitz J, Avorn J, Bohn R et al. Initiation of antihypertensive treatment during nonsteroidal anti-inflammatory drug therapy. *Journal of the American Medical Association.* 1994;272:781-786.

43. Anon. (Sanofi Pharmaceuticals, Inc.). Hyalgan package insert. 1997.

44. Anon. (Wyeth Laboratories). Synvisc package insert. 1997.

45. Chavez M. Glucosamine sulfate and chondroitin sulfates. *Hospital Pharmacy.* 1997;32(9):1275-1285.

Rheumatoid Arthritis in the Geriatric Patient

Leisa L. Marshall

SUMMARY. Rheumatoid arthritis (RA) is a systemic autoimmune disorder. Cartilage and bone destruction occur early in the disease. Although total remission is uncommon, therapy can slow the rate of disease progression. The majority of geriatric patients with RA developed the disease in mid-life, but some patients have elderly onset RA. Patients with elderly onset RA usually have a milder form of the disease than patients who develop RA earlier in life. Goals of therapy include controlling disease activity, slowing joint damage, decreasing pain and inflammation, and maintaining function for activities of daily living. Nonsteroidal anti-inflammatory drugs, corticosteroids, and disease modifying anti-rheumatic drugs (DMARDs) are the pharmacological agents most often used. DMARDs are now used earlier in the disease than in the past to control symptoms and to decrease joint destruction. The risks and benefits of therapy must be considered in developing a treatment plan for a geriatric patient. Geriatric patients are at increased risk for adverse effects from pharmacologic therapy compared to younger patients, and should be closely monitored for efficacy and toxicity. *[Article copies available for a fee from The Haworth Document Delivery Service: 1-800-342-9678. E-mail address: getinfo@haworthpressinc.com <Website: http://www.haworthpressinc.com>]*

KEYWORDS: rheumatoid arthritis, geriatric patients, nonsteroidal anti-inflammatory drugs, disease modifying anti-rheumatic drugs

---

Leisa L. Marshall, PharmD, CGP, is Clinical Assistant Professor, Mercer University Southern School of Pharmacy, Atlanta, GA 30341.

[Haworth co-indexing entry note]: "Rheumatoid Arthritis in the Geriatric Patient." Marshall, Leisa L. Co-published simultaneously in *Journal of Geriatric Drug Therapy* (Pharmaceutical Products Press, an imprint of The Haworth Press, Inc.) Vol. 12, No. 4, 1999, pp. 45-72; and: *Musculoskeletal Drug Therapy for Geriatric Patients* (ed: Marie A. Chisholm, and James W. Cooper) Pharmaceutical Products Press, an imprint of The Haworth Press, Inc., 1999, pp. 45-72. Single or multiple copies of this article are available for a fee from The Haworth Document Delivery Service [1-800-342-9678, 9:00 a.m. - 5:00 p.m. (EST). E-mail address: getinfo@haworthpressinc.com].

INTRODUCTION

Rheumatoid arthritis is a systemic, inflammatory, autoimmune disorder of unknown etiology.[1-3] Rheumatoid arthritis (RA) can result in disability, severe morbidity, and increased mortality.[2,4] Joint destruction occurs early in the disease.[5] Early diagnosis and introduction of appropriate therapy are imperative. Although therapy may slow joint destruction, it does not completely halt the progression of the disease.[2,6] The therapeutic regimens effective in slowing joint destruction and producing a partial remission are associated with side effects that often limit their use in geriatric patients.[6,7] Late onset disease may have a milder course, and respond to nonsteroidal anti-inflammatory drugs (NSAIDs) and less toxic disease-modifying anti-rheumatic drugs (DMARDs).[8] Geriatric patients with more severe disease may need combination therapy with multiple DMARDs.[8] Monitoring for efficacy and toxicity is imperative in the geriatric patient with active rheumatoid arthritis.

EPIDEMIOLOGY IN THE GERIATRIC POPULATION

RA affects approximately 1-3% of the adult population in the United States.[2,9] The incidence increases with age, and the prevalence is 2-3 times higher in females than males.[10] Although patients may develop RA as early as adolescence, onset is most common in patients age 40-60.[3] The incidence of RA in persons age 65 and older is higher than the general population from both RA with onset earlier in life and from patients newly diagnosed with RA in their 60s.[9]

ETIOLOGY

The etiology of RA is unknown. It is a systemic autoimmune disorder. Investigators believe that RA is induced by a variety of arthritogenic agents in genetically predisposed individuals.[11] Viruses or bacteria have been suspected to be the arthritogenic agents involved.[11] However, the presence of protein or messenger RNA for these infectious agents has yet to be found in the affected synovium.[12] Changes in the neuroendocrine hormones are believed to influence susceptibility and severity of the disease.[1] Symptom onset at menopause is common, and younger women often have reduced symptoms during pregnancy and increased symptoms in the postpartum period.[13] Rheumatoid arthritis is more common in women than men.

Genetic factors besides gender influence predisposition. Monozygotic twins and first-degree relatives of patients with rheumatoid arthritis have an increased incidence of developing the disease compared to the general population.[3,11] However, the majority of patients with RA do not have a first degree relative with the disease. Climate and place of residence have not been shown to significantly affect risk. Race is not a significant factor in disease development. Specific human leukocyte antigens have been associated with disease development and severity.[11]

PATHOPHYSIOLOGY

Rheumatoid arthritis is a systemic autoimmune disorder. In the affected joints of a patient with RA, synovial cells are injured through complex cell-cell interactions. A current theory is that antigen-presenting cells, triggered by an unknown stimulant, interact with specific receptors on T cells. Macrophages are then activated and the pro-inflammatory cytokines interleukin-1 and tumor necrosis factor alpha are secreted.[12] Another theory is that dendritic cells in the synovium are differentiated under the influence of cytokines released in response to nonspecific stimulation.[14] The dendritic cells then present autologous antigens to T cells. Cell types other than dendritic cells, for example, B cells or macrophages, may function as the antigen presenting cells.[12] Although RA has long been believed to be a T cell driven disease, other factors may be involved.[12,15] Most patients form antibodies termed rheumatoid factors.

The cells in the affected synovium become swollen and microvascular abnormalities develop. The synovium becomes edematous and hypertrophied as the disease progresses.[11] Inflammation occurs. Swelling and joint pain occur.[3] Abnormal cells destroy bone and cartilage where the bone and synovium attach.[11] With disease progression, the joint becomes deformed and unable to function as before. The inflammation and destruction cause the patient a great deal of pain and loss of functional ability. Total remission is uncommon in RA. If remission occurs, if is usually of brief duration.[16] Since cartilage and bone destruction occurs early in the disease, early diagnosis and therapy is imperative.[17]

CLINICAL MANIFESTATIONS

The onset of RA is often insidious, with the patient experiencing fatigue, weakness, low-grade fever, and stiffness and myalgias over several weeks to months.[18] Joint stiffness, pain, tenderness and swelling follow. Persistent swelling and pain of the joints is a hallmark of RA.[3] Morning stiffness may last over one hour. A few patients will present with a more acute onset of joint inflammation.

Joint involvement is usually symmetrical and of multiple joints. Large and small peripheral joints of the upper and lower extremities can be affected. The axial skeleton is not usually affected.[19] The most commonly involved joints are the small joints of the hands, wrists, and feet.[18] The proximal interphalangeal and metacarpophalangeal, but not the distal interphalangeal, joints of the hand and wrist are involved. The elbow, shoulder, hip, knee, and ankle joints may also be affected. With disease progression, the joints become deformed.

The majority of geriatric patients with RA developed the disorder in their fourth or fifth decade. They may have multiple joint deformities, and extra-articular complications, for example, rheumatoid nodules.[20] If the joints of the feet, ankles, and knees are involved, the resulting unsteady gait places the patient at an increased risk of falls. The patient may also have osteoporosis from use of corticosteroids to treat their disease. This increases their risk of fracture from injuries and falls.[21]

Some patients develop RA after age 60, which is termed elderly onset rheumatoid arthritis.[20] These patients usually have a milder form of the disease than those who develop symptoms earlier in life.[20] Patients with elderly onset RA experience fatigue, malaise, and a gradual onset of joint pain and stiffness. Multiple joints are affected.

RADIOGRAPHIC CHANGES AND LABORATORY STUDIES

Radiographs are used to determine the extent of joint space narrowing. Their primary purpose is to evaluate disease progression and the effectiveness of therapy.[3,4] Eventually, bony erosions and osteopenia occur at the affected joints. Magnetic resonance imaging may provide a more sensitive picture of joint changes, but is too expensive for routine use in patient evaluation.

Laboratory studies are used to help differentiate RA from other forms of arthritis. No one laboratory test is indicative for a definitive diagnosis, but typical findings in active RA include leukocytosis, thrombocytosis, and a mild anemia.[4] The erythrocyte sedimentation rate and C-reactive protein are usually elevated in active disease and may be monitored as an indicator of inflammation and the effectiveness of therapy. Abnormal amounts of rheumatoid factor in the serum are seen in approximately 85% of patients with rheumatoid arthritis.[22] Rheumatoid factor detects autoantibodies and may be elevated in other diseases, for example, sarcoidosis and tuberculosis. A positive rheumatoid factor in a patient with symptoms of rheumatoid arthritis is indicative of a more severe, unremitting case. Elderly onset RA patients who are negative for the rheumatoid factor often have a milder form of the disease.

CRITERIA FOR DIAGNOSIS

The American College of Rheumatology (then the American Rheumatism Association) last revised the criteria for diagnosis of RA in 1987. The seven criteria from 1987 are summarized below:

1. morning stiffness
2. arthritis of three or more joint areas
3. arthritis of hand joints
4. symmetric arthritis
5. rheumatoid nodules
6. serum rheumatoid factor
7. radiographic changes.[23]

For diagnostic purposes, morning stiffness, arthritis of three or more joint areas, arthritis of the hand joints, and symmetric arthritis must have been present for at least 6 weeks. A patient must meet four of the seven criteria to be definitively diagnosed.[23]

GOALS OF MANAGEMENT AND DESIGNING A TREATMENT PLAN

The goals of managing a geriatric patient with RA are the same as the goals for managing a younger patient: control disease activity, slow joint damage, alleviate pain, reduce joint inflammation, maintain function for activities of daily living, and maximize quality of life.[2,4] The majority of patients with rheumatoid factor positive, active disease affecting multiple joints develop joint damage or erosions within two years of disease onset.[2] Aggressive treatment may slow the progression of the disease in order to maintain the patient's quality of life. The rheumatologist will determine whether a geriatric patient has a milder or more severe form of the disease prior to making decisions about therapy. A careful history, review of systems, physical examination, documentation of symptoms, and baseline laboratory and radiographic studies should be done prior to designing a treatment plan.[2] Baseline laboratory tests needed include a complete blood count, platelet count, liver enzymes and a chemistry profile, including serum creatinine and blood urea nitrogen (BUN).[2] Serum rheumatoid factor, erythrocyte sedimentation rate, and C-reactive protein should be measured.[2]

The risks and benefits of therapy should be discussed with the patient. A geriatric patient who has had RA for years and now has little ongoing joint damage, or the geriatric patient with a mild form of elderly onset RA, will require less aggressive therapy than the geriatric patient with active ongoing joint destruction. The patient's general health status and co-morbid conditions will also influence the choice of therapy. In a patient who has had RA for years, therapy is based on response to current or prior therapy, as well as disease severity and progression. The therapeutic regimen will need to be continually reassessed for efficacy and toxicity in all patients with RA. Many patients discontinue therapy due to intolerable adverse effects. Diagnosis early in life, swelling of more than twenty joints, high levels of rheumatoid factor, elevated erythrocyte sedimentation rate, and the presence of extra-articular manifestations are each associated with more severe disease.[2]

NONPHARMACOLOGIC THERAPY

Nonpharmacologic therapy should be employed, in conjunction with pharmacologic therapy, for all patients with RA. The patient should be educated about the disease and resources available. Appropriate exercises, assistive devices, heat and cold treatments, and a proper nutritional program can benefit the patient. The patient should understand that the disease is long-term, and that several modes of therapy may be needed to improve symptoms. The patient, or patient's family, should contact the local chapter of the Arthritis Foundation. The national office of the Arthritis Foundation can be contacted at 1-800-283-7800 for information or to provide the patient with the location of a nearby office. The Arthritis Foundation publishes numerous pamphlets and books on many arthritic disorders. The Arthritis Foundation also has a useful web site: *www.arthritis.org* for patients or family members who prefer to access their information on-line.

A patient recently diagnosed with rheumatoid arthritis, or one having problems controlling symptoms, can benefit from a physical therapy consultation. Muscle atrophy, decreased muscle strength, and decreased flexibility can increase the functional decline in a patient. Exercise programs designed for RA patients have resulted in functional improvement without increasing joint inflammation.[4] Range-of-motion, isometric, isotonic, and aerobic exercises maintain range of motion, muscle strength, and patient endurance.[4,24] Certain exercises may need to be avoided during periods of acute inflammation, but even clinically active rheumatoid arthritis patients benefit from a well designed exercise program. Resting individual joints is usually recommended over total bed rest. However, most patients need an adequate amount of sleep at night, and usually benefit from several thirty-minute rest periods during the day.[6]

An occupational therapist should be consulted if a patient has joint deformity and decline in functional ability. Splints and orthoses may be needed to rest individual joints to manage pain, prevent contractures and preserve joint function.[6,24] An occupational therapist can also help the patient choose assistive devices for home activities of daily living.

A well balanced diet is recommended for patients. Adding special supplements, or eliminating certain foods from the diet, for example, red meat or diary products, has not been shown to affect symptoms.[4] Overweight patients should try to loose weight to decrease stress on the joints, and to avoid the development of osteoarthritis in weight-bearing joints.

THERAPEUTIC APPROACHES FOR PHARMACOLOGIC THERAPY

Background

There are numerous pharmacologic agents used in the management of RA. For many years, treatment of a newly diagnosed patient was based on a pyramid approach. Although the agents used in each level of the pyramid changed over the years, the basic concept behind the pyramid approach was the use of the least toxic agents first, followed by more toxic agents, if needed.[3] In the 1980s and 1990s rheumatologists began prescribing the more toxic agents earlier in the disease in an attempt to decrease the rapid joint destruction seen during the first few years after diagnosis.[6] Since joint destruction is rapid in the first few years after diagnosis compared to later in the disease process, early use of disease modifying anti-rheumatic drugs (DMARDs) is recommended to prevent disability.[25] Early use of DMARDs has the potential to reduce, and even prevent, joint damage.[2] Some rhematologists adopted a "sawtooth" strategy, and began prescribing a DMARD or combination of DMARDs soon after diagnosis to achieve symptom control.[26-28] Once the patient is placed on DMARD therapy, the physician evaluates the patient on a frequent basis for therapeutic efficacy and toxicity. If symptoms were not adequately controlled, the therapy looses efficacy, or the patient developed unacceptable adverse effects, another DMARD or combination of DMARDs would be prescribed.[26-28]

GUIDELINES OF THE AMERICAN COLLEGE OF RHEUMATOLOGY

In 1996 the American College of Rheumatology published "Guidelines for the management of rheumatoid arthritis."[2] These guidelines altered the traditional pyramid approach. The committee that developed these guidelines recognized that optimal management requires early diagnosis and appropriate use of medications that have that ability to reduce irreversible joint damage.[2] They recommended developing a longitudinal treatment plan for a newly diagnosed patient. The plan should be developed based upon the patient's prognosis and the potential risks and benefits of medications that are available. Appropriate consideration of all of the patient's problems and medication therapy is perhaps even more important in a geriatric patient than in a younger patient.

The guidelines emphasized that in newly diagnosed patients with active moderate to severe disease, aggressive therapy soon after diagnosis can slow the progression of joint damage.[2] The committee recommended initiation of treatment, after evaluation and diagnosis, with patient education, physical and occupational therapy, a NSAID for pain and swelling, and possibly local or oral steroids, depending on the patient. If the RA remains active after several weeks of this initial therapy, DMARDs should be used. This early use of DMARDs alters the traditional pyramid approach. In fact, the committee recommended using DMARDs within three months of diagnosis for patients who continue to have morning stiffness and pain, joint inflammation or pain, or elevation of erythrocyte sedimentation rate or C-reactive protein despite treatment with NSAIDs.[2] Patients with elderly onset RA, unlike patients with earlier onset severe disease, may achieve symptom control without using DMARDs or by using one of the less toxic DMARDs. Once a DMARD or DMARDs are prescribed, patients should continue to be evaluated for improvement, as a revised treatment plan may be needed. All patients should be counseled and monitored for side effects for all of the medications used for RA. The committee also developed "Guidelines for monitoring drug therapy in rheumatoid arthritis" which was published in 1996 as well.[7] Their recommendations for monitoring individual agents and specific side effects will be included in the sections that follow on each agent. Specific side effects will also be discussed later with each medication. The benefits of therapy should outweigh the side effects the patient experiences.

For patients unresponsive to or unable to tolerate medication therapy who develop structural joint damage, surgery should be considered. Hand, shoulder, knee, and hip surgeries can be very successful for RA patients.[2] A discussion of specific surgical procedures is beyond the scope of this review. However, a clinician caring for a patient recovering from restorative surgery should encourage the patient to make full use of the strategies, devices, and exercises recommended by the occupational and physical therapists. The patient will need their expertise and help to restore function in the affected joint.[2]

CURRENT THERAPEUTIC APPROACHES

Rheumatologists now advocate early use of a DMARD or combination of DMARDs for patients with active disease.[5,29] Although DMARDs are not completely successful in producing disease remission, they have been shown to reduce the rate of disease progression and formation of new destruction.[5] The use of DMARDs has also been shown to positively affect the short-term outcome of RA patients but the affect on long-term outcomes is still controversial.[25,28] RA patients with mild to severe disease benefit from DMARDs. There are differing opinions about which DMARD should be used first.[5] The rheumatologist will base this decision on medication safety and efficacy, the patient's disease activity and functional status, and the patient's other medical problems and therapy. DMARDs are slow acting, so a patient may not experience the full benefit from an agent for several months.[2] Often, a short course of an oral corticosteroid may be used until the DMARD becomes effective.[25]

If one DMARD does not produce an adequate response, a different DMARD should be prescribed. When necessary, combinations of two or more DMARDs with additive efficacy and differing side-effect profiles are used for patients with active moderate to severe disease.[6,25,30] Long-term DMARD therapy is problematic, as most individual DMARDs or combinations loose their effectiveness with time, or patients develop intolerable side effects. Only approximately 5-15% of patients who initially respond well to a DMARD will continue to benefit after 5 years.[28] Patients often discontinue therapy because of side effects.[26]

Combinations of DMARDs have been shown to slow disease progression more effectively than traditional therapy with a NSAID and one DMARD.[28,30] Successful DMARD combinations for adult RA patients include (1) methotrexate, sulfasalazine, and hydroxychloroquine, (2) sulfasalazine and hydroxychloroquine, (3) methotrexate and cyclosporine, and (4) gold and hydroxychloroquine.[6,29] An NSAID will be used with these combinations for control of pain and inflammation. A low-dose oral corticosteroid may also be prescribed on a short-term basis for some patients.[6,30] However, NSAIDs and oral prednisone have not been shown to reduce long term disability. The severity of RA, amount of disease progression, whether the disease is still active or under control, concomitant diseases and therapy, and efficacy and side-effect profiles of the agents used to treat RA must be carefully considered by the clinician prior to recommending therapy or changes in therapy.

SPECIFIC THERAPEUTIC ISSUES
FOR GERIATRIC PATIENTS

The majority of geriatric patients with RA developed the disease between the ages of 40 and 60.[3] Many already have joint deformities, and have a history of taking NSAIDs, corticosteroids, and DMARDs. If their disease is still active, they may require continuation of an NSAID and a DMARD or combination of DMARDs.[8] If disease activity has lessened, an NSAID, oral corticosteroid, and perhaps a less toxic DMARD may control symptoms. Geriatric patients commonly have concomitant illness and medication therapy that complicates the therapy for RA. Specific medications may be contraindicated in geriatric patients. Geriatric patients are also at increased risk of intolerable side effects. Furthermore, as previously mentioned, DMARDs are often not as effective long-term as they are in the first few (5 to 9) years of therapy.[26,28,30] The risks and benefits of therapy must be carefully considered in the geriatric patient.

Some patients over 65 with RA have elderly-onset RA. Patients with elderly onset RA are of two types: those with mild disease and those with severe disease who are positive for serum rheumatoid factor.[8] Nonpharmacologic therapy, NSAIDs, and possibly a low dose corticosteroid may satisfactorily control mild disease. If a DMARD is needed, an agent with low toxicity, i.e., hydroxychloroquine, may be used. Geriatric patients with elderly onset severe disease, similar to those with early onset active disease, will usually require other DMARDs or combinations of DMARDs to slow joint destruction.[8] The side effects and potential severe toxicity of the DMARDs limit their use in these patients. Patients may have contraindications for the use of these agents, or be unable to tolerate the adverse effects. Monitoring for safety and efficacy is vital for the geriatric patient with early or late onset RA. The usual doses, suggested monitoring parameters, and adverse effects of individual agents appear in Tables 2 and 3 and will be discussed below in the sections covering the different agents used.

PHARMACOLOGIC AGENTS

Nonsteroidal Anti-Inflammatory Drugs (NSAIDs)

NSAIDs reduce joint pain and swelling, but do not fully prevent joint damage and destruction, as described above. They are used for their analgesic and anti-inflammatory properties, and only rarely induce disease remission.[6] NSAIDs are used to control pain and inflammation in mild, moderate, and severe disease.[6] If used in comparable doses, the NSAIDs are similar in efficacy, but individual patient response to a particular NSAID may vary.[9] Table 1 in the article "Osteoarthritis in the Geriatric Patient" that appears in this volume has a complete list of commonly used NSAIDs, the doses recommended for geriatric patients with osteoarthritis, and suggestions for dosage reduction with mild renal impairment. The daily dosages recommended for rheumatoid arthritis are generally higher as higher dosages are required to produce anti-inflammatory effects than those required for analgesia. Table 1 of this paper lists example NSAIDs and dosages prescribed for geriatric patients with RA.[8,31] It is important to note that many geriatric patients are not able to tolerate these doses due to the increased incidence of side effects at anti-inflammatory doses.[4,8] Lower dosages should be prescribed initially, then increased if necessary. The patient should be monitored for adverse effects as the doses are increased. Daily dosages of NSAIDs should be decreased with declining renal function, and many NSAIDs are not recommended for use if patients have moderate to severe renal impairment.

A summary of adverse reactions and risk factors for adverse reac-

TABLE 1. Selective Nonsteroidal Anti-Inflammatory Drugs for Rheumatoid Arthritis

Medication	Recommended dosage for geriatric RA patients*
Diclofenac	25mg-50mg two to four times a day; or 100mg once a day of the extended release product
Etodolac	400mg two to three times a day
Fenoprofen	600mg three to four times a day
Ibuprofen	400mg to 600mg three to four times a day
Ketoprofen	75mg two to three times a day; or 200mg once a day of the extended release product
Nabumetone	500mg-1000mg once or twice a day
Naproxen	250mg-500mg twice a day
Oxaprozin	1200mg once a day
Sulindac	150mg-200mg twice a day

* Please note that these medications should be avoided in patients with moderate to severe renal impairment. Geriatric patients are at increased risk of adverse effects even with the recommended dosages. Patients should use the lowest dose possible that controls symptoms.
Sources: 8,31

tions to NSAIDs appears in Table 2 of the article "Osteoarthritis in the Geriatric Patient" in this volume. The text also contains a detailed description of the adverse reactions and suggested patient monitoring. Patients with certain concomitant diseases, for example hypertension or congestive heart failure, are at increased risk of developing adverse reactions to NSAIDs, and should only take NSAIDs if the benefits of therapy are greater than the risks. The text also contains a discussion of the medications that may be used concomitantly to prevent gastrointestinal adverse effects.

Of recent interest are the differences in selectivity of NSAIDs for two cyclooxygenase isoenzymes, cox-1 and cox-2. NSAIDs inhibit the conversion of arachidonic acid to intermediate and terminal prostaglandins, which are proinflammatory and work with other pain producing mechanisms. Cyclooxygenase is the specific converting enzyme which converts arachidonic acid to prostaglandins.[32] The cox-1 isoenzyme is produced continuously in the body and maintains the normal function of tissues in the body, including the kidney and gastrointestinal tract. In platelets it stimulates thromboxane induced platelet aggregation.[33,34] Inhibition of cox-1 can result in gastrointestinal ulceration and bleeding, reduced platelet aggregation and prolonged bleeding time, and decreased renal function. Production of the cox-2 isoenzyme is induced by stimuli.[35] The cox-2 isoenzyme produces prostaglandins in inflammation and mitogenesis.[32] A NSAID that inhibits cox-2 with little effect on cox-1 would have analgesic and anti-inflammatory properties with fewer side effects.

The majority of NSAIDs currently on the market preferentially inhibit cox-1 or have little selectivity for these isoenzymes.[33] Nabumetone and etodolac inhibit cox-2 to a greater degree than cox-1, but at therapeutic doses cox-1 inhibition occurs.[6] Indomethacin, piroxicam, and sulindac preferentially inhibit cox-1.[32] Fortunately, several new compounds selective for cox-2 are being studied in clinical trials or are being considered for approval by the Food and Drug Administration (FDA). Selective inhibitors of cox-2 have been found to have analgesic and anti-inflammatory effects without significantly decreasing gastric mucosal protection or renal perfusion.[33] Celecoxib, Rofecoxib, and Tenidap are examples of compounds under investigation or being reviewed by the FDA. Celecoxib and Rofecoxib were the first two selective cox-2 inhibitors to be considered for approval by the FDA. Both Celecoxib and Rofecoxib are expected to be available in

1999. In a four week, double blind, placebo controlled trial, celecoxib provided significant improvement in the signs and symptoms of RA.[35] The patients taking Celecoxib had significant improvement in morning stiffness, patient global assessment, and the number of painful and tender joints. No significant differences in adverse events were noted between the Celecoxib and placebo groups. A companion study evaluated Celecoxib's effect on cox-1 and cox-2. Healthy volunteers took 400mg twice a day (the highest dose that was used in the efficacy study) for seven days.[35] Platelet function was used to assess Celecoxib's possible effect on cox-1 since cox-1 inhibition decreases platelet aggregation. Platelet function was normal in the study group after seven days. It was determined that Celecoxib has no effect on cox-1 at doses of 400mg twice a day.

Selective cox-2 inhibitors would be beneficial for geriatric patients who need relief of pain and inflammation with a decreased risk of the usual side-effects associated with NSAIDs. Several other selective cox-2 inhibitors are under investigation in osteoarthritis and RA patients, so there will be four or five products to choose from in the near future.

Many geriatric patients may regularly take aspirin for cardiovascular prophylaxis. Patients taking aspirin and an NSAID, such as ibuprofen, are at increased risk of developing gastrointestinal ulceration. Since the cox-1 and cox-2 inhibitors also decrease platelet aggregation and increase bleeding time, the patient is at increased risk for gastrointestinal bleeding.[8] Once selective cox-2 inhibitors have been used for long periods of time in geriatric patients who are also taking aspirin for cardiovascular prophylaxis, it will be interesting to see if their risk of gastric ulceration and bleeding is significantly less than those taking an NSAID such as ibuprofen.

Disease Modifying Anti-Rheumatic Drugs (DMARDs)

The disease modifying anti-rheumatic drugs include azathioprine, cyclophosphamide, cyclosporine, gold, hydroxychloroquine, leflunomide, methotrexate, minocycline, penicillamine, and sulfasalazine. Table 2, "Doses and Adverse Effects of Selective Disease Modifying Anti-Rheumatic Drugs for RA in Geriatric Patients," gives the usual doses recommended for geriatric RA patients, and the most common adverse effects associated with the DMARDs.[2,6-8,20,25,31] Table 3, "Recommended Evaluation and Monitoring of Selective Disease Modifying Anti-Rheumatic Drugs," contains a summary of suggested baseline laboratory tests, and the follow-up laboratory and patient evaluation suggested for each agent.[6-8,20,25,31] Dosages, side effects, and monitoring will be discussed briefly in the text with each agent, since the information appears in Tables 2 and 3. It is important to note that the side effects and toxicities listed are those that have occurred in the adult population. Geriatric patients may be at increased risk of side effects and toxicities from the DMARDs due to their age, and concom-

TABLE 2. Doses and Adverse Effects of Selective Disease Modifying Anti-Rheumatic Drugs for RA in Geriatric Patients

Medication	Recommended dosage*	Adverse Effects*
Azathioprine	50mg q.d., increasing to a maximum of 50mg t.i.d.; decrease dose to 75% of above for Clcr of 10-50ml/min	GI symptoms, elevated LFTs, infrequent hepatotoxicity, infections, myelosuppression, lymphoproliferative disorders
Gold (oral)–Auranofin	3mg q.d., b.i.d., or t.i.d.	GI symptoms (especially diarrhea), rash, nephropathy, proteinuria, myelosuppression
Gold (parenteral)–Sodium aurothiomalate or aurothioglucose	Test dose of 5-10mg; increasing gradually to 50mg/week to a cumulative dose of 500-1000mg; decrease dose to 50mg every 2 weeks for the next 1000mg	Rash, stomatitis, nephropathy, proteinuria, myelosuppression, thrombocytopenia
Hydroxychloroquine	200mg b.i.d.; reduce to 200mg q.d. after response achieved	Infrequent rash, diarrhea, rare macular damage
Methotrexate (oral) Methotrexate (parenteral–I.M. or S.Q.)	5mg-7.5mg weekly; increase monthly by 2.5mg to 20mg weekly oral preferred; S.Q. less painful than I.M.	GI symptoms, stomatitis, infrequent hepatic fibrosis or cirrhosis, rare pulmonary infiltrates or fibrosis, myelosuppression
Minocycline	100mg b.i.d.	Photosensitivity, avoid in renal insufficiency; geriatric patients are at increased risk of dizziness, lightheadedness, and ataxia
Penicillamine	125mg-250mg q.d., increase gradually to 250mg t.i.d	Rash, stomatitis, glomerular nephritis, myelosuppression, rare autoimmune diseases
Sulfasalazine	500mg b.i.d.; increase gradually to 2gm per day in 2-4 divided doses	GI intolerance, photosensitivity, rash, rare Stevens Johnson syndrome, rare myelosuppression

* Clcr = Creatinine clearance, LFT = liver function test
Sources: [2,6-8,20,25,31]

TABLE 3. Recommended Evaluation and Monitoring of Selective Disease Modifying Anti-Rheumatic Drugs

Medication	Baseline laboratory evaluation	Routine laboratory evaluation	Patient evaluation
Azathioprine	CBC, platelets, creatinine, AST, ALT	CBC & platelets q 1-2 weeks initially & with dosage changes, then q 1-3 months; AST/ALT q month initially then q 1-2 months	Symptoms of myelosuppression*
Gold (oral)– Auranofin	CBC, platelets, urine for protein	CBC, platelets, urine for protein q 4-12 weeks	Symptoms of myelosuppression, edema, rash, diarrhea
Gold (parenteral)– Sodium aurothiomalate or aurothioglucose	CBC, platelets, creatinine, urine for protein	CBC, platelets, urine for protein q 1-2 weeks for 20 weeks, then prior to each injection	Symptoms of myelosuppression, edema, rash, oral ulcers, diarrhea
Hydroxychloroquine	CBC, creatinine, AST/ALT	CBC, creatinine, AST/ALT q 6 months	Eye examination at baseline and q 6 months for visual changes, funduscopic and visual fields
Methotrexate	CBC, Hepatitis screen, AST/ALT, alkaline phosphatase, albumin, creatinine, chest X-ray within past year	CBC, platelets, AST/ALT, albumin, creatinine q month	Symptoms of myelosuppression, lung function, lymph node swelling, nausea or vomiting, stomatitis, rash
Minocycline	CBC	CBC q 6 months	
Penicillamine	CBC, platelets, creatinine, urine for protein	CBC, urine for protein q 2 weeks until dosage stable, then q month	Symptoms of myelosuppression, edema, rash
Sulfasalazine	CBC, AST/ALT	CBC, AST/ALT q 2 weeks initially, then q month	Symptoms of myelosuppression, photosensitivity, rash

Sources: [6-8, 25, 31]
* symptoms of myelosuppression (bone marrow suppression)–fever, increased bruising and bleeding, infections, anemia

itant illness and medication therapy.[9] Most studies in the literature describe the use of particular DMARDs or combinations in middle-aged, not elderly, adults.[8] In the geriatric RA patient appropriate monitoring is essential. The suggested monitoring and evaluation that appear on Table 3 are based primarily on the "Guidelines for monitoring drug therapy in rheumatoid arthritis" developed by the American

College of Rheumatology and published in 1996 and selective references discussing medication therapy for geriatric RA patients.[7,8] The DMARDs are relatively slow in onset, with patients not experiencing the full benefit of therapy for several weeks to months.

Azathioprine

Azathoprine is a purine analog used for moderate to severe RA, when other DMARDs have failed to provide adequate control of the disease.[7,8,25] Relative contraindications for its use include renal insufficiency or liver disease.[3] Azathioprine's efficacy and toxicity has not been reported in the literature in geriatric patients sufficiently to assess any differences between the efficacy and toxicity in younger patients.[8] Azathioprine can cause myelosuppression with the doses used for RA. Patients at increased risk for myelosuppression include individuals also taking angiotensin converting enzyme inhibitors or allopurinol, and individuals with renal insufficiency.[7] Since many geriatric patients have some degree of renal insufficiency, they are at increased risk and should be monitored closely. The most common side effect of azathioprine is gastrointestinal intolerance, which causes about 10% of treated patients to discontinue therapy.[7]

Cyclophosphamide

Cyclophosphamide is an alkylating agent that is effective for RA, but not often used due to the severe adverse effects, i.e., hemorrhagic cystitis, carcinogenesis, leukopenia, associated with its use.[25] It is rarely prescribed for geriatric patients, and should only be used in severe active RA with severe extraarticular complications unresponsive to other DMARDs.[8]

Cyclosporine

Cyclosporine has been effective in several studies of RA patients, and a few of these studies included some geriatric patients with RA.[8,25] However, cyclosporine's side-effect profile limits its use to severe progressive RA patients when other DMARDs have not been effective.[25] It can cause renal failure that can be irreversible. Geriatric patients were at an increased risk of renal failure compared to younger patients in the few studies of cyclosporine that included geriatric patients.[8] Any individual with hypertension, pre-existing renal insufficiency, or taking a NSAID is at increased risk of renal toxicity from cyclosporine.[8] Cyclosporine should not be used in patients with a creatinine clearance below 80ml/minute, which precludes its use in most geriatric patients.[8]

Gold

Gold is available as oral and parenteral formulations. Although serious toxicity from oral gold is rare, it is not very effective as a sole DMARD. Oral gold is used in mild RA, often in combination with other DMARDs.[25] One recent two-year double-blind placebo controlled trial of elderly onset RA patients compared therapy with auranofin 3mg bid to placebo.[36] Oral prednisolone was used for intolerable joint pain and stiffness in both the auranofin and placebo patients. The RA patients who received the auranofin consumed significantly less prednisolone over the study period than those who were taking the placebo. The auranofin group also had a greater decrease in joint pain, but the decrease in the number of swollen joints was similar in the auranofin group and the placebo group. Diarrhea and other gastrointestinal side effects were the most common adverse events reported in both the auranofin and placebo group. In fact, gastrointestinal side effects, especially diarrhea, are common with oral gold therapy and a common reason for discontinuing therapy.

Parenteral gold preparations are clinically more effective than oral gold. Parenteral gold preparations have been used in RA for 50 years.[8] At present, they are usually a choice after several other DMARDs have been tried unsuccessfully.[6] Patients have had short-term and intermediate control of symptoms and even disease remission with parenteral gold. Approximately 60-80% of RA patients respond to parenteral gold therapy, but approximately 35% of RA patients discontinue the injections due to side-effects.[6] A test dose of 5 to 10mg should be used initially, followed by a gradual increase to a weekly dose of 50mg. Most patients experience symptom control after a cumulative dose of 500mg to 1000mg.[8] Once the patient's symptoms are under control, the dose is tapered to 50mg every other week for the next 1000mg. At this time, dosage frequency should be decreased to every three to four weeks.[8]

The efficacy and toxicity of parenteral gold does not appear to be influenced by age.[8] If patients are closely monitored, the rate of severe toxicity is low. However, many patients will experience skin rashes and oral ulcers as side effects. Urinalysis and complete blood counts must be checked prior to injections to monitor for nephropathy and bone marrow suppression. Geriatric patients will need to be counseled about the necessity of frequent laboratory monitoring for side effects. They, or the nurses or pharmacists involved in their care, should also understand the importance of contacting the physician if they develop a rash, mouth ulcers, blood in the urine, bleeding, or other problems while on gold therapy.

Hydroxychloroquine

Hydroxychloroquine is often one of the first DMARDs used, especially for mild RA, as it is one of the least toxic DMARDs. Efficacy in geriatric patients is similar to efficacy in younger patients.[8] In one study 46% of RA patients who had the elderly onset rheumatoid factor positive disease responded positively to hydroxychloroquine therapy.[37] However, hydroxychloroquine is usually not effective as the sole DMARD in severe RA.[25] Hydroxychloroquine is also often used in combination with other DMARDs for mild, moderate, or severe disease.[6] Hydroxychloroquine has been successfully combined with sulfasalazine or methotrexate, and with both sulfasalazine and methotrexate.[38,39]

A recent study of middle-aged patients with active RA compared maintenance therapy with (1) placebo with methotrexate as needed for disease flare, (2) hydroxychloroquine, and (3) hydroxychloroquine with methotrexate as needed for disease flare.[39] Maintenance therapy was initiated after an initial treatment period in which all patients had received both hydroxychloroquine 400mg per day and methotrexate 7.5mg-15mg per week for 24 weeks. Disease variables improved significantly in all three groups during the initial treatment period with both medications. With maintenance therapy, the median time to disease flare was 62 days in the placebo plus methotrexate for flare group, 285 days in the hydoxychloroquine group, and 90 days in the hydroxychloroquine plus methotrexate for flare group. The authors concluded that the combination of hydroxychloroquine and methotrexate was effective, and that maintenance hydroxychloroquine may extend the response to the combination therapy. Of interest to the geriatric patient was the similarity in adverse effects during the combination and maintenance therapy periods and the low discontinuation rates. Only 5% of patients discontinued the combination therapy because of clinical or laboratory adverse effects. The toxicities of hydroxychloroquine and methotrexate were not additive.[39]

Leflunomide

Leflunomide was FDA approved for adults with RA in late 1998. Leflunomide, which inhibits pyrimidine synthesis, has both immunosuppressant and anti-inflammatory effects.[40] The dosage approved for RA is 10mg per day for three days, followed by 20mg per day.[41] The dosage may be lowered to 10mg per day if 20mg per day results in intolerable side effects.

In placebo-controlled trials of varying doses, leflunomide improved patient global assessment and the number and intensity of swollen and tender joints.[40] Most patients in these trials had been treated with several other DMARDs previously. Patients were allowed to remain on NSAIDs and oral steroids, if necessary. The patients who received leflunomide 10 and 25mg per day had an increased clinical response compared to patients who received 5mg per day. However, 25mg per day increased the incidence of adverse effects, so 20mg per day was the high-end dose used in later studies. The patients taking 5mg per day responded only slightly better than those on placebo.

Leflunomide 20mg per day was compared to methotrexate therapy and to sulfasalazine therapy in several separate studies.[42] Leflunomide, methotrexate, and sulfasalazine reduced disease progression when used individually in these studies. Leflunomide was similar in efficacy to methotrexate, and more effective than sulfasalazine.[42]

The most common leflunomide side effects reported in clinical trials were diarrhea, rash, alopecia, and elevated liver enzymes.[40,43] Nephrotoxicity and bone marrow suppression were not reported, but leflunomide is not recommended for use in patients with severe immunodeficiency.[40,42] Leflunomide is also not recommended for patients with hepatic impairment. Liver enzyme tests should be monitored closely in all patients. Leflunomide is carcinogenic and teratogenic in animals. Leflunomide has not been studied and used sufficiently in geriatric patients to provide specific dosage and monitoring recommendations, and additional cautions for use. It should only be used after other safer agents failed to control the disease.

Methotrexate

Over the last ten years, methotrexate has become the most widely prescribed DMARD for adults with RA. It is often used as the initial DMARD when a patient has severe disease, and as an alternative or additional agent in moderate disease. Methotrexate has become the most often prescribed DMARD because of its predictable benefits, high efficacy to toxicity ratio, and rapid onset of action compared to other DMARDs.[2,6,8,44,45] Over 50% of all patients prescribed methotrexate remain on the medication with good results after three years of therapy, which is longer than the continuation rate with other DMARDs.[2,26] For other DMARDs most patients have discontinued therapy because of side effects or unsatisfactory control of disease at three years of therapy.[45] Methotrexate has been beneficial to RA patients in several long-term studies of three to ten year duration.[45] Methotrexate has also been effective in reducing symptoms in approximately 89% of geriatric patients with elderly-onset RA.[37] However, methotrexate does not produce complete remission in the majority of patients.[45] It has been shown to slow the progression of joint erosions to a greater degree than most other DMARDs, but not to halt the disease progression.[45]

The initial dose in geriatric patients is 5mg-7.5mg once weekly. Oral methotrexate is preferred for patient convenience.[45] The dose is increased monthly by 2.5mg to a maximum dose of 20mg weekly.[31] Some rheumatologists will use 25-30mg weekly, if necessary. Patients usually respond after one to two months of therapy, and continue to have an increased response before plateau at three to four months.[26] If the patient does not achieve symptom control with oral therapy, parenteral therapy may be used as absorption is more predictable.[45] The dose may need to be decreased, but should still be given weekly. Subcutaneous injection is preferred over intra-muscular injection as the intra-muscular injection is quite painful.

Side effects, life-threatening toxicities, and recommended patient evaluation and monitoring appear on Tables 2 and 3. The most common side effects from methotrexate are gastrointestinal. Patients may develop mucositis, nausea, vomiting, and diarrhea. Mild alopecia can occur. Concomitant use of folic acid 1mg daily can decrease these side-effects, as they may be due to folic acid depletion.[7] This low dose of folic acid will not decrease the effectiveness of the methotrexate.[25] Folic acid supplementation also decreases the risk of hematologic toxicity.[7]

Liver disease can occur, especially if a patient has pre-existing liver problems.[8] Pre-existing liver disease is a relative contraindication for methotrexate use. Other risk factors for liver toxicity include age, duration of therapy, and alcohol ingestion.[7] Patients should not drink alcohol while taking methotrexate. Since the risk of liver toxicity is low in patients without pre-existing liver impairment, the American College of Rheumatology guidelines advise liver biopsy only in cases when patients have elevated liver enzymes that persist during or after therapy.[7] Liver enzymes should be routinely monitored in all patients.

Other than liver disease and alcohol abuse, relative contraindications for use include significant pulmonary disease, bone marrow suppression, and renal impairment.[2] Methotrexate can cause a rare hypersensitivity pneumonitis in 3-5% of patients.[25] Patients with pulmonary disease may be at greater risk of developing the hypersensitivity pneumonitis. Hematologic toxicity is rare at the doses used for RA.[4] Patients with folate deficiency, taking another antifolate agent, i.e., trimethoprim, or with renal impairment are considered to be at increased risk for hematologic toxicity.[7] Therefore, methotrexate may be more toxic in geriatric patients with mildly impaired renal function.[8] The dosage of methotrexate should be decreased in geriatric patients with renal impairment, since methotrexate is 90% eliminated through the kidney.[31] Both NSAIDs and salicylates can decrease methotrexate's clearance, which is one reason why low doses of methotrexate are used initially, to assess patient response. Methotrexate is contraindicated in patients with severe renal or hepatic impairment or pre-existing blood dyscrasia or bone marrow suppression.[31]

Minocycline

Minocycline is a tetracycline analog that has been used with limited success in younger patients with early mild to moderate disease.[6,46] There are few severe toxicities associated with its use. However, minocycline can cause lightheadedness, dizziness, and vertigo. Geriatric patients are at increased risk of experiencing these side-effects. The full benefit of minocycline therapy does not occur until approximately one year of therapy. Minocycline is not FDA approved for RA, but it may be a safe agent to use in elderly onset RA.

Penicillamine

Penicillamine is effective for RA, but it is not commonly used because of its side-effect profile and inconvenient dosing schedule. Penicillamine has similar efficacy to gold or sulfasalazine with increased toxicity compared to these agents.[3] It is equally effective in geriatric and younger patients, but geriatric patients have an increased incidence of adverse effects compared to younger patients.[8] Common adverse effects associated with penicillamine use for RA include skin rash, stomatitis, and dysgeusia. Rare, but severe, adverse effects of penicillamine include thrombocytopenia and nephropathy.[7] Penicillamine use has also induced several autoimmune disorders, i.e., myasthenia gravis, systemic lupus erythematosus, polymyositis, and Goodpasture's syndrome. It should be discontinued if the patient develops an adverse effect suspected to be caused by penicillamine.

Sulfasalazine

Sulfasalazine is an effective agent for early treatment of mild to moderate cases of RA. It is effective in decreasing the symptoms of patients with elderly onset RA. Both the efficacy and toxicity are similar in geriatric and younger patients with RA.[8] Sulfasalazine is the most often used DMARD in Europe.[6] In the U.S., sulfasalazine is often used with hydroxychloroquine in mild to moderate disease, or with hydroxychloroquine and methotrexate in moderate to severe disease.[6]

The starting dose of sulfasalazine is 500mg twice a day with food, increasing to two to at most three grams per day, in divided doses.[8,25] The medication should be taken with meals to decrease gastrointestinal upset. Patients may experience benefits from therapy within two months. Sulfasalazine should not be given to patients who are allergic to salicylates or sulfa drugs.[6,31] Common side effects include nausea, vomiting, headache, photosensitivity, rash, and fever. The major, but rare, toxicities associated with sulfasalazine are bone marrow suppression, nephrotoxicity, hepatitis, and severe rashes.[3] Hematologic adverse effects include leukopenia, thrombocytopenia, hemolysis, agranulocytosis, and aplastic anemia. Toxic epidermal necrolysis, Stevens-Johnson syndrome, and exfoliative dermatitis have occurred in patients taking sulfasalazine.[3] Patients should be advised to report any rashes that develop. Appropriate laboratory monitoring should detect hematologic toxicites in order to discontinue therapy.

Corticosteroids

Corticosteroids effectively suppress inflammation and relieve symptoms in active RA, but prolonged use is not recommended due to adverse effects associated with extensive use of high doses.[2] Corticosteroids have been indicated for use in RA for many years. Most patients who have taken oral corticosteroids for RA have continued to experience progressive joint deformities despite symptom relief.[2,25] There is some evidence that corticosteroids may decrease the rate of joint damage.[25]

Prednisone is the oral corticosteroid recommended for RA, with a usual dose of 5 to 10mg per day.[2] If prednisone is used, the dose should be adjusted to the lowest possible dose to help control symptoms. Long term use at doses above 10mg per day is not recommended.[2] Prednisone may be used to decrease symptoms and disease activity when initiating or adjusting DMARD therapy or during a period of disease flare.[2] It could also be used when NSAIDs and trial of combination DMARDs have failed to adequately control the disease.[2]

Patients with elderly onset RA have responded well to low dose short term prednisone use. Geriatric patients have also experienced symptom relief with short-term high dose therapy for unremitting disease.[8] However, the adverse effects of long term use or short term high dose therapy present a greater problem in geriatric patients than in a younger population.[8] These adverse effects include sodium and water retention, hypokalemia, hypertension, hyperglycemia, osteoporosis, and an increased infection rate.[8]

Local injections of corticosteroids are also highly effective in relieving symptoms in specific joints.[2] Injecting the involved joints without changing the prescribed DMARD therapy can treat disease flares affecting a few joints. A joint should not be injected more than once in a three month time period.[2] Intra-articular injections are considered a safe and effective procedure if used in this manner. More frequent injections may lead to further cartilage degeneration.[8] Frequent disease flares or uncontrolled symptoms in multiple joints are usually an indication that the DMARD therapy needs modification.

BIOLOGICAL RESPONSE MODIFIER

Etanercept

Etanercept is a biological response modifier recently FDA approved for the reduction of the signs and symptoms of moderate to severe active RA for patients who have failed to respond adequately to DMARDs. It is also approved for use in combination with methotrexate for patients who have not responded adequately to methotrexate alone. The dosage approved is 25mg subcutaneously twice a week. Patients may continue taking NSAIDs, corticosteroids, analgesics, and methotrexate while on etanercept.[47]

Etanercept is a recombinant tumor necrosis factor receptor that binds and neutralizes tumor necrosis factor's biological activity. Tumor necrosis factor is one of the cytokines causing the inflammation and resultant joint damage in RA.[47] Increased levels of tumor necrosis factor occur in the synovial fluid and plasma of patients with active RA.[48] Antagonism of tumor necrosis factor decreases disease activity in some patients.[48]

In a multicenter, randomized double-blind placebo-controlled trial comparing three different doses of etanercept to placebo, patients who received etanercept had improvement in signs and symptoms of RA.[48] A dose response curve was observed, with the patients who received the highest dose, 16mg per square meter of body surface area, experiencing the most significant improvement. Patients included in the study all had been unsuccessfully treated with between one and four DMARDs. They were allowed to remain on stable doses of NSAIDs and a corticosteroid throughout the study period, but must have discontinued any other DMARD at least four weeks prior to the study period. The mean age of the study participants was 53 years, and 77% of these patients had had RA for more than 5 years. The medication was well tolerated, with only one study patient discontinuing therapy, because of a mild injection site reaction. In fact, the most common adverse events were these mild injection site reactions. A few patients developed transient mild respiratory tract symptoms. No laboratory abnormalities developed.

Several other Phase II, III, and open label trials have been conducted. All found etanercept to be safe and effective in RA patients who had failed treatment with DMARDs.[47,49] About 100 patients 65 years old or older were included in the various clinical trials.[47] No significant differences in response or safety between these patients and younger patients were observed.[47] The manufacturer cautions that geriatric patients may yet prove to be more sensitive to the effects of etanercept.[47]

CONCLUSION

Geriatric patients may have elderly onset RA or earlier onset RA on long-standing duration. Therapy must be tailored to the patient's signs and symptoms. Consideration of the patient's other medical problems and medication therapy is imperative. The goals of therapy are to relieve pain, decrease inflammation, slow joint damage, maintain joint integrity, and preserve the patient's functional ability as much as possible. Although pharmacologic regimens may control symptoms and decrease joint damage, these regimens are unable to produce complete remission over a long period of time.

REFERENCES

1. Wilder R. Rheumatoid arthritis: epidemiology, pathology, and pathogenesis. In: Schumacher H, ed. *Primer on the Rheumatic Diseases.* 10th ed. Atlanta, Georgia: Arthritis Foundation; 1993:86-89.

2. Guidelines of the American College of Rheumatology ad hoc committee on clinical guidelines. Guidelines for the management of rheumatoid arthritis. *Arthritis and Rheumatism.* 1996;39(5):713-722.

3. Sperling R. Rheumatoid Arthritis. In: Carlson K, Eisenstat S, eds. *Primary Care of Women.* St. Louis: Mosby; 1995:179-190.

4. Semble E. Rheumatoid arthritis: new approaches for its evaluation and management. *Arch Phys Med Rehabil.* 1995;76:190-201.

5. Weinblatt M. Rheumatoid arthritis: treat now, not later! *Annals of Internal Medicine.* 1996;124(8):773-774.

6. Gremillion R, vanVollenhoven R. Rheumatoid arthritis: designing and implementing a treatment plan. *Postgraduate Medicine.* 1998;103(2):103-123.

7. Guidelines of the American College of Rheumatology ad hoc committee on clinical guidelines. Guidelines for monitoring drug therapy in rheumatoid arthritis. *Arthritis and Rheumatism.* 1996;39(5):723-731.

8. Nesher G, Moore T. Recommendations for drug therapy of rheumatoid arthritis in elderly patients. *Clin Immunother.* 1996;5(5):341-350.

9. Nesher G, Moore T. Rheumatoid arthritis in the aged. *Drugs & Aging.* 1993;3(6):487-501.

10. Lawrence R, Helmick C, Arnett F et al. Estimates of the prevalence of arthritis and selected muscoloskeletal disorders in the United States. *Arthritis and Rheumatism.* 1998;41(5):778-799.

11. Goronzy J, Weyand C. Rheumatoid arthritis: epidemiology, pathology, and pathogenesis. In: Klippel J, ed. *Primer on the Rheumatic Diseases.* 11th ed. Atlanta, GA: Arthritis Foundation; 1997:155-160.

12. Arend W. The pathophysiology and treatment of rheumatoid arthritis. *Arthritis and Rheumatism.* 1997;40(4):595-597.

13. Goemaere S, Ackerman C, Goethals K et al. Onset of symptoms of rheumatoid arthritis in relation to age, sex, and menopause transition. *Journal of Rheumatology.* 1990;17:1620-1622.

14. Thomas R, Lipsky P. Presentation of self peptides by denditric cells: possible implications for the pathogenesis of rheumatoid arthritis. *Arthritis and Rheumatism.* 1996;39:183-190.

15. Schiff M. Emerging treatments for rheumatoid arthritis. *American Journal of Medicine.* 1997;102(suppl 1A):11S-15S.

16. Wolfe F. The natural history of rheumatoid arthritis. *Journal of Rheumatology.* 1996;23(suppl 44):13-22.

17. Pope R. Rheumatoid arthritis: pathogenesis and early recognition. *American Journal of Medicine.* 1996;100(suppl 2A):3S-9S.

18. Schuna A, Schmidt M, Walbrandt D. Rheumatoid arthritis and the seronegative spondyloathropathies. In: DiPiro J, Talbert R, Yee G et al., eds. *Pharmacotherapy: a pathophysiologic approach.* 3rd ed. Stamford: Appleton and Lange; 1997:1717-1733.

19. Fan P. A focus on musculoskeletal complaints in the elderly patient. *Family Practice Recertification.* 1998;20(3):21-55.

20. Nesher G, Moore T. Clinical presentation and treatment of arthritis in the aged. In: Perry H, ed. *Clinics in Geriatric Medicine: the aging skeleton.* Vol. 10. Philadelphia: W.B. Saunders; 1994:659-675.

21. Miller-Blair D, Robbins D. Rheumatoid arthritis: new science, new treatment. *Geriatrics.* 1993;48(6):28-38.

22. Anderson R. Rheumatoid arthritis: clinical and laboratory features. In: Klippel J, ed. *Primer on the Rheumatic Diseases.* 11th ed. Atlanta, GA: Arthritis Foundation; 1997:161-167.

23. Arnett F, Edworthy S, Bloch D et al. The American Rheumatism Association 1987 revised criteria for the classification of rheumatoid arthritis. *Arthritis and Rheumatism.* 1988;31:315-324.

24. Ross C. A comparison of osteoarthritis and rheumatoid arthritis: diagnosis and treatment. *The Nurse Practitioner.* 1997;22(9):20-39.

25. Paget S. Rheumatoid arthritis: treatment. In: Klippel J, ed. *Primer on the Rheumatic Diseases.* 11 ed. Atlanta: Arthritis Foundation; 1997:168-174.

26. Blackburn W. Management of osteoarthritis and rheumatoid arthritis: prospects and possibilities. *American Journal of Medicine.* 1996;100(suppl 2A):24S-30S.

27. Fries J. Reevaluating the therapeutic approach to rheumatoid arthritis: the "sawtooth" strategy. *Journal of Rheumatology.* 1990;17(suppl 22):12-15.

28. Mottonen T, Paimela L, Ahonen J et al. Outcome in patients with early rheumatoid arthritis treated according to the "sawtooth" strategy. *Arthritis and Rheumatism.* 1996;39(6):996-1005.

29. Wilske K, Yocum D. Consensus statement: Rheumatoid arthritis: the status and future of combination therapy. *Journal of Rheumatology.* 1996;23(suppl 44):110.

30. Brooks P. Recent advances: Rheumatology. *British Medical Journal.* 1998;316:1810-1812.

31. Semla T, Beizer J, Higbee M, eds. *Geriatric Dosage Handbook.* 3rd ed. Hudson, OH: Lexi-Comp; 1997.

32. Polisson R. Nonsteroidal anti-inflammatory drugs: practical and theoretical considerations in their selection. *The American Journal of Medicine.* 1996;100(2A):31S-36S.

33. Badger A, Lee J. Advances in antiarthritic therapeutics. *Drug Discovery Today.* 1997;2(10):427-435.

34. Cryer B, Feldman M. Cyclooxygenase-1 and cyclooxygenase-2 selectivity of widely used nonsteroidal anti-inflammatory drugs. *American Journal of Medicine.* 1998;104(5):413-21.

35. Lipsky P, Isakson P. Outcome of specific cox-2 inhibition in rheumatoid arthritis. *Journal of Rheumatology.* 1997;24(suppl 49):9-14.

36. Glennas A, Kvien T, Andrup O et al. Auranofin is safe and superior to placebo in elderly-onset rheumatoid arthritis. *British Journal of Rheumatology.* 1997;36(8):870-877.

37. Lance N, Curran J. Late-onset, seropositive erosive rheumatoid arthritis. *Semin Arthritis Rheum.* 1993;23:177-182.

38. O'Dell J, Haire C, Erikson N et al. Treatment of rheumatoid arthritis with methotrexate alone, sulfasalazine and hydroxychloroquine, or a combination of all three medications. *New England Journal of Medicine.* 1996;334(20):1287-1291.

39. Clegg D, Dietz F, Duffy J et al. Safety and efficacy of hydroxychloroquine as maintenance therapy for rheumatoid arthritis after combination therapy with methotrexate and hydroxychloroquine. *Journal of Rheumatology.* 1997;24(10):1896-1902.

40. Plosker G, Wagstaff A. Leflunomide. *Clin Immunother.* 1996;Oct 6(4):300-305.

41. M Abramowicz et al. New drugs for rheumatoid arthritis. *The Medical Letter.* 1998;40(1040):110-111.

42. Anonymous. (Hoechst Marion Roussel). Package literature for Arava. 1998 September.

43. Rozman B. Clinical experience with leflunomide in rheumatoid arthritis. *Journal of Rheumatology.* 1998;25(suppl 53):27-32.

44. Kremer J. Historical overview of the treatment of rheumatoid arthritis with an emphasis on methotrexate. *Journal of Rheumatology.* 1996;23(suppl 44):34-37.

45. O'Dell J. Methotrexate use in rheumatoid arthritis. In: Cash J, ed. *Rheumatic Disease Clinics of North America.* Vol. 23. Philadelphia: WB Saunders; 1997:779-793.

46. O'Dell J, Haire C, Palmer W et al. Treatment of early rheumatoid arthritis with minocycline or placebo: results of a randomized, double-blind, placebo-controlled trial. *Arthritis Rheum.* 1997;40(5):842-848.

47. Anon. (Immunex Corporation). Etanercept package literature. 1998 November.

48. Moreland L, Baumgartner S, Schiff M, Tindall E et al. Treatment of rheumatoid arthritis with a recombinant human tumor necrosis factor receptor (p75)-Fc fusion protein. *New England Journal of Medicine.* 1997;337(3):141-147.

49. Weinblatt M, Moreland L, Schiff M et al. Long-term and phase III treatment of DMARD-failing rheumatoid arthritis patients with TNF receptor p75 Fc fusion protein-Abstract 572. *Arthritis and Rheumatism.* 1997;40(suppl):S126.

Managing Hyperuricemia and Gout in the Geriatric Patient

William E. Wade
James W. Cooper

SUMMARY. Hyperuricemia and gout in the elderly are common problems that should be anticipated and treated differently than in younger persons. The risks of NSAIDs, intravenous (IV) and oral colchicine are reviewed. Intraarrticular or systemic steroids may be preferable to NSAIDs for treatment of acute gout in the elderly who have a history of NSAID or low-dose aspirin usage or NSAID gastropathy. Since 90% of primary gout is due to underexcretion of urate, allopurinol in doses adjusted for creatinine clearance is the preferred therapy for prophylaxis of gouty attacks. Uricosuric drugs such as probenecid and sulfinpyrazone are usually not indicated since less than 10% of primary gout is due to uric acid overproduction, and the renal function of most elderly also may contraindicate the use of these medications. Drug classes such as thiazide diuretics, low-dose aspirin and alcohol use may predispose the elderly to gout. Asymptomatic hyperuricemia treatment is not indicated in the absence of gout damage to the heart, kidney, or musculoskeletal systems. *[Article copies available for a fee from The Haworth Document Delivery Service: 1-800-342-9678. E-mail address: getinfo@haworthpress inc.com <Website: http://www.haworthpressinc.com>]*

KEYWORDS: gout, elderly, hyperuricemia

William E. Wade, PharmD, is Associate Professor and James W. Cooper, PhD, is Professor, College of Pharmacy, University of Georgia, Athens, GA 30602-2354.

Address correspondence to: James W. Cooper, College of Pharmacy, University of Georgia, Athens, GA 30602-2354.

[Haworth co-indexing entry note]: "Managing Hyperuricemia and Gout in the Geriatric Patient." Wade, William E., and James W. Cooper. Co-published simultaneously in *Journal of Geriatric Drug Therapy* (Pharmaceutical Products Press, an imprint of The Haworth Press, Inc.) Vol. 12, No. 4, 1999, pp. 73-86; and: *Musculoskeletal Drug Therapy for Geriatric Patients* (ed: Marie A. Chisholm, and James W. Cooper) Pharmaceutical Products Press, an imprint of The Haworth Press, Inc., 1999, pp. 73-86. Single or multiple copies of this article are available for a fee from The Haworth Document Delivery Service [1-800-342-9678, 9:00 a.m. - 5:00 p.m. (EST). E-mail address: getinfo@haworthpressinc.com].

DEFINITIONS AND EPIDEMIOLOGY

Hyperuricemia and gout occur as a consequence of some abnormality in either the production or excretion of uric acid, or both. Primary gout is more than 90% due to uric acid renal underexcretion, with less than 10% due to uric acid overproduction. Secondary gout can occur from uric acid overproduction due to purine dietary excess or enzyme defects, increased nucleotide turnover and alcohol abuse. Other secondary causes of gout from renal underexcretion of uric acid include renal failure, and acidosis primarily due to drug use.[1,2]

Gout and hyperuricemia are associated with a strong male preponderance and peak incidence in middle age. Yet, both hyperuricemia and gout can and often do persist as an individual ages. Post-menopausal women approach the same prevalence as men. Hyperuricemia may be an asymptomatic disorder with elevated serum uric levels being the only manifestation. By definition, hyperuricemia is the serum uric acid level that leads to physiological supersaturation of uric acid. This value is generally considered to be in excess of 7.0 mg/dL for men and 6.0 mg/dL for women. Men tend to become hyperuricemic in their third decade, while women usually develop this condition only after menopause. Asymptomatic hyperuricemia is present in about 5% of adults and 10% of insitutionalized patients.[2]

Gout occurs with deposition of monosodium urate crystals in and around the joints, heart, cartilage and kidneys. Generally, many years of hyperuricemia are necessary to allow for the formation of crystals and microtophi in connective tissues, producing the inflammation associated with gout. Men usually develop gout in their mid 40s, following 10 to 20 years of hyperuricemia. Women who develop gout following menopause do so only after many more years, such that gout in women is a disease of the more elderly woman in her 60s to 70s. Only 5 to 17% of gouty subjects are women. Premenopausal gout is rare and seems to occur only in women with a strong family history of this disorder. Uric acid nephrolithiasis occurs in 10 to 15% of patients with gout. Overall, gout has a prevalence of approximately 1% in the population. Increasing lifespan and the use of low-dose aspirin for stroke and myocardial infarction prevention as well as thiazide diuretics for high blood pressure and congetstive heart failure is expected to increase the prevalence of gout especially in the elderly.[1-3]

The relationship between hyperuricemia and untreated gout involves two or three overlapping phases that may take 20 to 40 years to occur: a usually lengthy phase of asymptomatic hyperuricemia; acute to recurrent gouty attacks separated by relatively asymptomatic intervals; and finally approximately one in ten persons will develop chronic tophaceous gouty arthritis.[14,15]

PATHOPHYSIOLOGY

Uric acid is the end product of purine metabolism, has no useful function, and is considered a waste product. The normal uric acid pool in humans is approximately 1,200 mg, while patients with gout may have a urate pool of 18,000 to 31,000 mg. Endogenous purine sources are derived from 3 primary sources: diet, nucleic acid conversion and *de novo* biosynthesis. Several enzyme systems are responsible for regulating purine metabolism. Abnormalities in these enzyme systems may result in an overproduction of uric acid. Additionally, myeloproliferative and lymphoproliferative disorders (such as lymphocytic leukemias, multiple myeloma, certain solid lymphomas) are associated with increased nucleic acid breakdown which may increase the uric acid concentration found in the blood and tissues.[1-7]

Uric acid excretion occurs through both the urine and gastrointestinal (GI) tract, with most urate/uric acid appearing in the urine. However, in the presence of declining renal function, the amount of urate/uric acid excreted in the GI tract increases several fold.

Factors contributing to decreased urinary elimination of uric acid include a functional reduction in glomerular filtration with aging (please see Cockcroft-Gault Formula in Table 1; the [140-age] function represents this functional loss), defects in tubular secretion of urate, competition with urate for tubular secretory sites, and low urine pH.[1-4] The functional loss of creatinine clearance (CrCl) should be taken into account, along with organic changes in renal function in the elderly patient. The Cockcroft-Gault equation for estimating CrCl should be an integral part of the pharmacotherapeutic planning for the elderly.[8] Based on a 282 elderly patient study, a reasonable approximation of 40 ml/min. can be made for most elderly, pending the results of a serum creatinine.[9] Table 1 depicts expected laboratory values and the CrCl estimation equation.

In patients with declining renal function, the amount of uric acid excreted in the GI tract increases several fold. Conditions which may

TABLE 1. Laboratory Findings in Hyperuricemia and Gout [1-4,6,7]

Lab Study	Normal Range[1]	Possible Significance of Abnormal Results
Serum Uric Acid		Elevated values represent hyperuricemia which may
males	3-7 mg/dL	lead to gout
females	3-6 mg/dL	

Target Level of Treatment = 4-6 mg/dL

Serum Creatinine (Cr)		Elevated values suggest renal impairment
males	0.5-1.5 mg/dL	
females	0.5-1.5 mg/dL	

Cr Clearance (CrCl) = 140 − age × body weight (kg.)/Serum Cr × 72
(males; females × 0.85; always round Cr < 1.0 to 1.0) (ref. 8)

24-hour Urine Uric Acid	up to 750 mg	Elevated values suggest patient is an overproducer of uric acid
Urine Uric Acid/Creatinine Ratio	up to 75%	Values greater than 75% suggest patient is an overproducer of uric acid

[1] Normal values may vary among laboratories

be associated with hyperuricemia and gout include pernicious anemia, obesity, congestive heart failure, diabetic ketoacidosis, starvation, acute alcoholism, hyperlipidemia, hyper- and hypoparathyroidism, hypothyroidism, and osteoarthritis. In elderly men, gout is commonly associated with high blood pressure, obesity and alcohol abuse. High blood pressure is present in approximately 30 to 70% of patients with gout and is associated with a reduced renal clearance of uric acid. Obese individuals have been shown to have an increased urate production as well as a decline in renal clearance of uric acid. Alcohol exerts a dual effect on urate metabolism in that it decreases renal excretion of urate and increases catabolism of purine nucleotides. As a consequence, elevated uric acid pools develop.[1-7] Gout attacks occur in chronic alcoholics at lower serum urate levels than in nonalcoholics: a recent study of acute gout attacks found that the index serum urate for alcoholics was 7.7 ± 1.3 mg/dL for 15 alcoholics and 10.1 ± 1.3 mg/dL for 34 nonalcoholics (p < 0.01).[10]

As previously stated, gout in the female population tends to occur only in postmenopausal women. This is thought to be due to the effects of estrogens on the uric acid pool. Estrogens increase tubular excretion of uric acid. Most women with gout have high blood pressure which results in mild renal insufficiency and are receiving diuretic therapy. Ethanol abuse and obesity are not usually contributing factors in elderly females. Chronic use of several medications may contribute to elevated serum uric acid levels in these patients. These drugs include diuretics, especially hydrochlorothiazide in doses of 25 mg or more per day or thaizide equivalents, pyrazinamide, nicotinic acid, levodopa, ethambutol, cytotoxic agents, low dose salicylates (less than 2 grams per day), pancreatic extracts and vitamin B-12 injections.[1-7]

DIAGNOSIS

Gout in the elderly is generally indistinguishable from that found in younger subjects. However, the geriatric patient is more likely to have chronic gout with unremitting inflammation, attacks in multiple joints, gout associated with diuretic therapy and acute onset gout associated with trauma or other illnesses. For example, acute arthritis, most commonly gouty, may affect as many as one of seven stroke patients on the paretic side and markedly impair their rehabiliation and functional recovery.[11] Additionally, gout in females most typically is seen in those who are 75 years of age or older. Although one would prefer making the diagnosis empirically based on symptomatology, a definitive diagnosis can only be made upon needle aspiration and visualization of mono-sodium urate crystals under polarized light microscopy.

The presentation of gout in older patients can be quite varied and may mimic other arthritic disorders. Most elderly patients have osteoarthritis as their underlying musculoskeletal disease, and may be self-medicating with salicylates or NSAIDs. Because treatment of these disorders differs, it is essential to confirm the diagnosis of gout by arthrocentesis.[1-3]

Although useful in making the diagnosis of hyperuricemia, serum uric acid values are of no use in differentiating acute gout from other inflammatory disorders. Reasons for this include the fact that many elderly patients are hyperuricemic, but only a small minority will ever have gout. Additionally, 40% of elderly patients experiencing an acute attack of gout will have a normal serum uric acid level at the time of their attack. Another laboratory test which may be useful in making a definitive diagnosis is the 24-hour urine collection for uric acid. Excretion of greater than 750 mg uric acid in 24 hours on a regular diet suggests that a patient may be an overproducer of purines. A urine uric acid/creatinine ratio can be performed from a single urine specimen, and values greater than 75% suggest overproduction of purines. The use of thiazide diuretics in doses of 25 mg of hydrochlorothiazide or more per day for high blood pressure or congestive heart failure and the presence of functional renal impairment also increase the likelihood of the need for antigout therapy.[12,13]

TREATMENT

Non-Pharmacologic

Obesity increases endogenous urate production resulting in elevated serum uric acid levels. Thus, weight reduction in obese individuals is desirable. Avoidance of alcohol consumption will decrease the frequency of gout. Finally, preventing injury to joints affected with tophi will minimize the risk of the patient experiencing an acute exacerbation of gout. This step may involve simple measures such as avoiding tight fitting shoes or high heels. Although purine-restricted diets theoretically would lower uric acid production, these diets are unpalatable, difficult to adhere to and of questionable efficacy.[1-8]

Acute Gout Pharmacotherapy

NSAIDs

Special care must be taken to use anti-gout drugs wisely. Appropriate consideration for each agent's pharmacology and benefit/risk ratio should be given and therapy must be individualized for each patient. With an acute onset of gout, the goal of therapy is to treat the inflammation with early aggressive therapy. This can be accomplished with nonsteroidal anti-inflammatory agents, colchicine, or with corticosteroids. Nonsteroidals are generally considered the drugs of choice in most patients with acute gout, however the risk of these agents in the elderly is greater and must be used cautiously, especially if low-dose aspirin is assumed to be used by the elderly. Common NSAID adverse drug effects include anemia, gastritis or ulcerations and/or bleeding of the mucosa of the GI tract, epigastric pain, dyspepsia and nausea.[16]

NSAIDs are the drug class most commonly involved in adverse drug reaction (ADR) hospitalization of the elderly from the nursing home as well as the community setting.[17] NSAID therapy without gastroprotection may cost $200 per patient per month of NSAID usage. NSAIDs used without misoprostol or a proton pump inhibitor may produce as much as 20% fatality rate per year of unprotected NSAID usage.[18] In the short term usage of NSAIDs fewer than 10% of patients across all age groups have been found to have serious toxicity leading to drug withdrawal.[2]

Nonsteroidal anti-inflammatory agents have also been shown to induce renal syndromes, including papillary necrosis, nephrotic syndrome, acute renal failure and interstitial nephritis.[19] The consumption of NSAIDs, especially those with longer-halves, has recently been linked to the development of functional renal impairment in elderly who had prior renal disease, hyperuricemia or gout.[20] If an NSAID is used it should be for no more than 1 to 3 days. Gastro-protection with antacids or omeprazole should be considered for that 1 to 3 day period or longer. NSAIDs are generally better tolerated than colchicine and NSAIDs may produce a response even when used late in the attack.[2] In the presence of high blood pressure, congestive heart failure, renal or hepatic impairment and especially in those with a history of GI bleeding, NSAIDs are absolutely contraindicated.[2]

Colchicine

Colchicine is used to interrupt the inflammatory response in acute gout. Two-thirds of patients will respond to colchicine therapy if initiated within the first day of the onset of gouty symptoms. Unfortunately, 80% of patients experience gastrointestinal toxicity of nausea, abdominal pain and diarrhea and many patients do not seek care for an acute gout attack within 24 hours.[21] The recommended dose of colchicine is 0.3 to 0.6 mg orally every hour until the relief of symptoms is experienced, not exceeding 2 to 3 mg per day or until the patient develops diarrhea. Common side effects patients are likely to experience from this drug include hyperperistalsis, nausea, vomiting, abdominal cramping and or diarrhea. Intravenous (IV) colchicine, in a dose of 1 to 2 mg per 24 hours, can be administered in younger patients unable to tolerate oral colchicine or nonsteroidal anti-inflammatory compounds. However, IV colchicine should not be routinely administered in the elderly since renal, hepatic and/or heart failure as well as arrhythmias (e.g., atrial fibrillation) are risk factors commonly found in the elderly which predispose one to colchicine toxicity.[2] A recent study documented that IV colchicine is commonly misprescribed, and called for prescriber education if IV colchicine is to be used in any patient population.[22]

Corticosteroids

Corticosteroids may also interrupt the inflammatory response in acute gout. Elderly patients experiencing an acute attack of gout are commonly encountered who are not candidates for NSAIDs due to the aforementioned concurrent drug use and/or history of conditions in which NSAIDs should not be used. Oral, intraarticular (IA), intramuscular (IM) or IV corticosteroids can be used in the treatment of acute mono- or polyarticular gout in elderly patients with renal failure, peptic ulcer, hepatic impairment, congestive heart failure, high blood pressure or other conditions contraindicating the use of NSAIDs.[2,23] An alternative to corticosteroids is adrenocorticotropic hormone (ACTH) in a dose of 40 to 80 units intramuscularly every 6 to 12 hours for one to three days. A recent study compared single doses of ACTH 40 IU with 60mg of triamcinolone acetonide (TA) IM in acute gouty arthritis and found fewer patients receiving TA needed a second injection based on patient response.[24] These findings suggest that ACTH may be less preferable than corticosteroids for acute gout. If ACTH is used rather than corticosteroids the likelihood of re-visit may be increased.

Post-Acute Gout Attack Considerations

Once an acute attack of gout has been adequately controlled, it is necessary to determine if long term therapy is necessary. Not all patients that experience one attack will experience another; or many years may elapse prior to another acute episode. Thus the decision to initiate chronic therapy is often based upon the number of acute attacks experienced, serum uric acid level, patient compliance, and whether the patient has a positive family history for gout.

Treatment options include "as needed" (P.R.N.) therapy, long-term suppressive therapy, or hypouricemic therpy. P.R.N. therapy consists of the use of colchicine or nonsteroidal anti-inflammatory agents at the first sign of the onset of an acute attack. The same precaution mentioned earlier for colchicine and NSAIDs in acute attacks should be recalled. Neither drug class is usually indicated and short-term corticosteroids are generally again preferred. Long-term suppressive therapy constitutes daily low doses of a NSAID (e.g., sulindac 200 mg B.I.D.) or colchicine 0.6 mg once or twice a day. Both drugs have their risks and neither drug affects the hyperuricemia nor progression to topaceous lesions.

Additionally long-term use of colchcine can lead to neuromyopathy, myelotoxicity, alopecia and malabsorption syndrome.[25] Colchicine myopathy may present after as long as 7 years of chronic daily low-dose usage.[26]

Chronic Gout Pharmacotherapy

Allopurinol

Several options are available to the clinician based on frequency of gout attacks, presence of elevated uric acid, and/or tophaceous deposits development. Fewer than 10% of elderly patients with gout are over-producers of uric acid; most (> 90%) are underexcretors of uric acid.[2] The drug of choice for underexceretion of uric acid in gout is allopurinol. Allopurinol is preferred for elderly patient, especially patients with tophi, renal insufficiency (assumed to present in all elderly on a functional loss basis) or nephrolithiasis. Allopurinol is a xanthine oxidase inhibitor which prevents the conversion of hypoxanthine to xanthine and xanthine to uric acid. Allopurinol undergoes metabolism to oxypurinol, which is also an inhibitor of xanthine oxidase and has a half-life of 14 to 26 hours. Allopurinol can be administered in once daily doses of 100 to 600 mg. It is recommended to begin with 50 to 100 mg daily in the elderly. The dose is increased until the desired serum uric acid level is achieved and based on the estimated creatinine clearance (Table 1). Dosage adjustment is necessary in renal impairment. Table 2 lists recommended doses with declining renal function. Side effects associated with allopurinol include skin rash (especially with co-administration of ampicillin or amoxicillin), toxic epidermal necrolysis, systemic vasculitis, bone marrow suppression and renal failure. The skin rash seen in about 2% of recipients is apparently an immunologic reaction to the drug. This rash can progress to an allopurinol hypersensitivity syndrome to include fever, eosinophilia, leukocytosis, worsened renal function and hepatocellular injury in less than 0.5% of allopurinol recipients. Death has been reported to occur in approximately 28% of patients experiencing this hypersensitivity reaction.[26,27]

Allopurinol should never be initiated in an acute attack of gout since this agent may further worsen the condition and possibly

TABLE 2. Dosage Adjustment of Allopurinol in Declining Renal Function[2]

Creatinine Clearance (ml/min)	Maintenance Dose
80	250 mg daily
60	200 mg daily
40	150 mg daily
20	100 mg daily
10	100 mg Q O D
0	100 mg Q 3 days

precipitate episodes in other joints. Once the acute episode is resolved allopurinol therapy is initiated for the prevention of further acute attacks. Should this be undertaken, it is suggested that colchicine prophylaxis in the dose of 0.6 mg once to twice daily be given initially or a short-term corticosteroid with quick taper (e.g., prednisone at successive daily doses 20 mg, 15 mg, 10 mg and 5 mg). Allopurinol should be introduced in a dose of 50 to 100 mg daily and increased at 2 to 4 week intervals by 50 to 100 mg per day, according to the creatinine clearance estimated from table 1 and dose in Table 2 or until the serum uric acid level falls below 4 mg/dL. Long term therapy of gout following the first acute attack is usually not necessary since many elderly will not experience further attacks and allopurinol therapy can result in a greater risk of side effects than the risk of a further gout attack. Some recommend more than 4 severe attacks of gout within a year, but most would start allopurinol after the second attack within a year.[2]

If allopurinol is utilized, the goal of therapy is to lower serum uric acid levels to the point that monosodium urate crystals dissolve. At 37 degrees centigrade body temperature, this usually occurs at uric acid levels less than 4 mg/dL. Colchicine prophylaxis in a dose of 0.6 mg one to two times daily or an NSAID for a week or more is often necessary upon initiation of allopurinol therapy. Colchicine or NSAID therapy may need to be continued for as long as several weeks after an acute attack to prevent an acute exacerbation of gout.

Discontinuation of allopurinol is followed by a rapid increase in uric acid, but acute attacks may not occur for prolonged periods of time after discontinuation. Oxypurinol has been shown to be effective in those with a history of allopurinol hypersensitivity, but cross-allergic reactions can occur.[29]

Other Urate-Lowering Drugs

Probenecid and sulfinpyrazone act by interfering with the tubular reabsorption of filtered urate in the kidney. The recommended dose of probenecid is 250 mg to 0.5 g daily for 1 to 2 weeks, then 500 mg BID up to 1.5 grams daily, in divided doses. Since probenecid raises urinary uric acid levels, increased fluid consumption is a must in patients receiving probenecid to prevent urate nephropathy and nephrolithiasis. However, probenecid is not effective in patients with a glomerular filtration rate of less than 80 ml/min. Unfortunately, most elderly patients have creatinine clearances less than 50 to 80 ml/min.[9]

Sulfinpyrazone is a potent uricosuric agent; however, this drug shares many of the same toxic bone marrow effects as its parent compound, phenylbutazone. The recommended dose of sulfinpyrazone is 50 to 100 mg BID for 1 to 2 weeks, then 100 to 200 mg BID up to 400 mg BID (800 mg daily), with most patients requiring 300 to 400 mg per day. Because sulfinpyrazone reduces platelet function and has a potential benefit in protecting against acute myocardial infarction and recurrent venous thrombosis, it may be a preferred uricosuric agent. However, as with probenecid, sulfinpyrazone is not recommended nor effective in patients with declining renal function (CrCl < 50 ml/min) and may have a greater likelihood to cause ADRs in renal impairment. Since sulfinpyrazone is related to phenylbutazone and due to the expected functional renal impairment in the elderly, sulfinpyazone is a poor choice for urate lowering in the elderly.[30]

Aspirin has uricosuric properties when given in large doses (i.e., over 4 grams daily), yet this dose is impractical and produces salicylate toxicity in many older patients.[31,32] In elderly patients with rheumatoid arthritis, salicylate toxcity appears more commonly than in younger patients, even at lower mean doses in older (39.1 ± 2.4 mg/kg/day) than in younger patients (49.8 ± 3.9 mg/kg/day).[33] Low dose salicylate therapy (< 2 grams/day) can precipitate acute gout attacks by preventing tubular excretion of uric acid.

Not all salicylates cause problems with uric acid levels. A salicylic acid derivative, diflunisal, has mild uricosuric properties and may be useful in patients with osteoarthritis and gout. The recommended dose of this compound is 500 mg twice daily.[34]

DRUG-INDUCED HYPERURICEMIA

Asymptomatic hyperuricemia may occur in up to 65 to 75% of elderly patients receiving low-dose aspirin, a thiazide, or pyrazinamide. Serum uric acid retention begins soon after a diuretic is introduced and an average increase in serum uric acid concentration between 1.2 and 1.5 mg/dL is usually seen. This change in uric acid levels may or may not be dose-related. Fortunately, few patients with asymptomatic hyperuricemia develop gout. Studies suggest only 1 to 2% of elderly patients with elevated serum uric acid levels progress to symptomatic gout. The likelihood of an individual developing gout is proportional to the degree and duration of hyperuricemia and is less than the likelihood of an adverse reaction to hypouricemic therapy. Generally speaking, an interval of 20 to 25 years or longer following the development of hyperuricemia will elapse before gout will appear. With diuretic-induced hyperuricemia, this interval is somewhat shorter, but may be in terms of years. Medications known to produce hyperuricemia may need to be discontinued, decreased in dose or changed to other medications if possible. For example, a thiazide in doses of 25 mg per day or more may be reduced to less than 25 mg per day if renal function and fluid retention status permit; or the thiazide can be changed to an angiotensin converting enzyme inhibitor (ACEI). Low-dose aspirin at 40 to 160 mg per day may not present as significant a challenge to tubular secretion competition as doses of 325 to 2,000 mg aspirin; the benefit of low-dose aspirin in myocardial infarction and stroke prevention suggests that all clinicians should assume that low-dose aspirin is in use until denied by the patient. Finally, a recent study confirmed an earlier suspected effect of long-term allopurinol therapy; a higher risk for the development of cataracts.[35] Thus, the general consensus is not to treat all patients with asymptomatic hyperuricemia with drugs which may produce significant side effects to prevent a small fraction from developing an acute attack of gout. After all, acute gout, although painful, is not a serious disorder and can easily be managed once present.[1-4,6,7]

CONCLUSION

The treatment of acute and chronic gout has been reviewed. Relief of pain and inflammation are the goals of acute gout treatment, and center on corticosteroids and minimal usage of NSAIDs and colchicine. Chronic gout may need to be treated with allopurinol adjusted to estimated creatinine clearance, depending on the number of attacks one suffers and the uric acid level. Probenecid and sulfinpyrazone are rarely indicated due to diminished renal function, lack of efficacy and excessive adverse drug reactions. Long-term NSAIDs and colchicine are generally avoided due to unacceptable toxicity. Whether to treat asymptomatic hyperuricemia, avoidance of hyperuricemia drugs in those with a history of gout and guidelines for uric acid lowering are also presented.

REFERENCES

1. Campbell SM. Gout: How presentation, diagnosis and treatment differ in the elderly. Geriatrics. 1988; 43:71-77.

2. Fam AG. Gout in the elderly. Drugs & Aging 1998;13(3):229-243.

3. Doherty N, Dieppe P. Crystal deposition disease in the elderly. Clin Rheum Dis 1986; 12:97-116.

4. Reginato AJ, Schumacher HR. Crystal-associated arthropathies. Clin Geriatr Med 1988; 4:295-322.

5. Wallace SL, Singer JZ. Review: systemic toxicity associated with intravenous administration of colchicine–guidelines for use. J Rheumatol 1988; 15:495-9.

6. Roubenoff, R. Gout and hyperuricemia. Rheum Dis Clin North Am 1990; 16:539-50.

7. Wallace SL, Singer JZ. Therapy in gout. Rheum Dis Clin North Am 1988; 14:441-57.

8. Cockcroft DW, Gault MH. Prediction of creatinine clearance from serum creatinine. Nephron 1976;16:31-41.

9. Cooper JW. Renal function assessment in nursing home patients. A prospective 6-month study in 282 patients. J Geriat Drug Ther 1991; 5(3):59-72.

10. Vandenberg MK, Moxley G, Breitbach SA et al. Gout attacks in chronic alcoholics occur at lower serum urate levels than in nonalcoholics. J Rheumatol 1994; 21;700-704.

11. Chakravarty K, Durkin CJ, al-Hillawl AH et al. The incidence of acute arthritis in stroke patients, and its impact on rehabilitation. Q J Med 1993;86:819-823.

12. Gurwitz JH, Kalish SC, Bohn RL et al. Thiazide diuretics and the initiation of anti-gout therapy. J Clin Epidemiol 1997; 50:953-959.

13. Scott JT, Higgens CS. Diuretic-induced gout: a multifactorial condition. Ann Rheum Dis 1992;51:259-261.

14. Ross GA, Seegmiller JE. Hyperuricemia and gout:classification, complications and management. N Engl J Med 1979;300:1459-1468.

15. Becker MA. Clincial aspects of monosodium urate monohydrate crystal deposition disease gout. Rheum Dis Clin North Am 1988; 14:377-394.

16. Cooper JW. Consultant pharmacist effect on NSAID costs and gastropathy over a 5-year period. Consult Pharm 1997; 12:792-796.

17. Cooper JW. Adverse drug related hospitalizations of nursing facility patients: a 4-year study. Sou Med J, in press.

18. Cooper JW, Wade WE. Pharmacist intervention in NSAID therapy in a geriatric nursing facility: a 1-year study, abstract no. 209, ACCP 1998 Annual meeting.

19. American Hospital Formulary Service-Drug Information–1998, p. 1600.

20. Henry D, Page J, Whyte I et al. Consumption of NSAIDs and the development of functional renal impairment in elderly subjects. Results of a case-control study. Br J Clin Pharmacol 1997; 44: 85-90.

21. Ahern MJ, Rid C, Gorton TP et al. Does colchicine work? The results of the first controlled study in acute gout. Aust NZ Med 1987; 17:301-304.

22. Evans TI, Wheeler MT, Small RE et al. A comprehensive investigation of in-patient intravenous colchicine use shows more education is needed. J Rheumatol 1996; 23:143-148.

23. Fam AG. Current therapy of acute microcrystallinea arthritis and the role of corticosteroids. J Clin Rhematol 1997; 3:35-40.

24. Siegel LB, Alloway JA, Nashel DJ. Comparison of ACTH and traimcinolone in hte treatment of acute gouty arthritis. J Rheumatol 1994; 21:1325-1327.

25. Kunel RW, Duncan G, Watson D et al. Colchcine myopathy and neuropathy. N Engl J Med 1987; 316:1562-1568.

26. Tapal MF. Colchcine myopathy. Scand J Rheumatol 1996; 25:1050106.

27. Hande KR, Noone RM, Stone WJ. Severe allopurinol toxicity:description and guidelines for prevention in patients with renal insufficiency. Am J Med 1984; 76:47-56.

28. Murrell GAC, Rapeport WG. Clinial pharmacokinetics of allopurinol. Clin Pharmacokinet 1986;11:343-353.

29. Walter-Sack I, de Vries JX, Viau AT et al. Uric acid lowering of effect of oxy-purinol sodium in hyperuricemic patient-therapeutic equivalence to allopurinol. J Rhematol 1996;23:498-501.

30. Facts and Comparisons–1998, Lippincott, St. Louis, p. 1518.

31. Gittleman DK. Chronic salicyalte intoxication. Sou Med J 1993;86:683-685.

32. Durnas C, Cusack BJ. Salicylate intoxication in the edlerly. Recognition and recommendations on how to prevent it. Drug Aging 1992;2:20-34.

33. Girgor RR, Spitz PW, Furst DE. Salicylate toxicity in elderly patients with rheumatoid arthritis. J Rheumatol 1987; 14:60-66.

34. Facts and Comparisons–1998, Lippincott, St. Louis, p. 1463.

35. Garbe E. et al. Exposure to allopurinol and the risk of cataract extraction in elderly patients. Arch Opthalmol 1998; 116:1652-1656.

Index

Page numbers followed by *f* indicate figures; those followed by *t* indicate tables.